THE DOCTOR OF THE FUTURE IS HERE

THE DOCTOR OF THE FUTURE IS HERE

True health care is preventative,
True prevention is generational.

By Dr. Raj Jheeta, ND

Published in Canada by Generational Health First, Inc.
Copyright © 2014 by Dr. Raj Jheeta and Michael H. Hanson

www.drjheeta.com and www.generationalhealthfirst.com
Library and Archives Canada Cataloguing in Publication

Jheeta, Raj—1961
The Doctor of the Future is Here, Take Back Control of Your Health / Generational Health First / The 3 P's / The Three E's – Education, Evaluation and Empowerment / Dr. Jheeta's Algorithm, created by Dr. Raj Jheeta, ND, with Michael H. Hanson.

Includes bibliographical references.
Includes; Glossary
ISBN 978-0-9918442-1-0
1. Health—Prevention   2. Health—Naturopathic Medicine   3. Health—Self-Help   4. Health—Family and Children   5. Health—Anti-Aging

Printed and bound in Canada

Table of Contents

Author's Notes 1

INTRODUCTION 3

PART I: EDUCATION..16

Introduction To Informed Consent 17

Chapter 1: How Do We Learn From the Past? 19

Chapter 2: How – and Why – Did Food Become Fast?................ 28

Chapter 3: How Did Drugs Become Such a Big Part of Health? 35

Chapter 4: How Did We Lose Control of Our Body Composition?...... 44

Chapter 5: How Did We Develop Food Intolerances?................ 58

Chapter 6: How Did Stress Take Over Our Lives? 69

Chapter 7: How Has Toxic Load Become a Health Issue? 76

Chapter 8: Can We Control the Aging Process?........................ 84

Chapter 9: How Did We Lose Control of Our Children's Health?........ 92

Chapter 10: What Is Generational Health First?....................... 102

PART II: EVALUATION 111

Introduction.. 112

Chapter 11: Dr. Jheeta's Algorithm... 114

Chapter 12: Body Composition Evaluation.............................. 119

Chapter 13: Food Intolerance Evaluation................................ 122

Chapter 14: Stress Evaluation 125

Chapter 15: Toxic Load Evaluation 128

Chapter 16: Wellness or Age-Management Evaluation 131

Chapter 17: Dr. Jheeta's Algorithm for Children..................... 133

Chapter 18: Specialized Health Care.. 135

PART III: EMPOWERMENT 137

Introduction... 138

Chapter 19: Take Control of Body Composition 140

Chapter 20: Take Control of Food Intolerances..................... 158

Chapter 21: Take Control of Stress 168

Chapter 22: Take Control of Toxic Load................................... 182

Chapter 23: Take Control of Aging 190

Chapter 24: Take Control of Your Child's Health 202

Chapter 25: Take Control of Health Care................................. 216

Conclusion 223

Sources.. 228

About the Author 244

GLOSSARY.. 245

AUTHOR'S NOTES

WRITING NOTES

This book is a work of non-fiction. Anecdotes refer primarily to cases in the author's practice, supplemented by a few stories from acquaintances. I have changed identifying details to protect the privacy of those depicted. Health and treatment related details are recalled from memory. I have used imaginary "dialogue" in these stories to present sometimes-dry information in an entertaining way. Occasionally, when an issue is complex or simply dry, I have engaged in imaginary question-and-answer "conversations" with a "reader." These passages do not represent real conversations with real people. Finally, to avoid a perception of gender bias, I have alternated between masculine and feminine pronouns.

USE OF EVIDENCE

Naturopathic and allopathic care differs in that the primary goal of naturopathic care is to assist the healing power of nature and prevent disease while the primary goal of allopathic care is to treat signs and symptoms of disease. These differences mean naturopathic and allopathic doctors can practice medicine and perform research differently. Naturopathic doctors draw on a large pool of traditional knowledge, a small but growing pool of recent naturopathic research, and some aspects of allopathic research. Allopathic researchers and practitioners have highly developed methods and a large body of scientific research, and often consider naturopathic methods and evidence, or naturopathic use of allopathic evidence, inherently less reliable than allopathic methods and evidence.

One of my goals in writing this book is to increase efforts between the two disciplines to work side by side and learn from each other, thereby providing patients with a broad spectrum of care. To that end, I have sought to support my words with research from a variety of sources – traditional, allopathic, and naturopathic. I firmly believe history and experience show neither allopathic nor naturopathic medicine can be as effective alone as they can together. However, I will be the first to say that some of the ideas in this book

1

cannot stand up to allopathic scrutiny because they were not developed for allopathic purposes. They must be accepted on their own merits or not at all.

DISCLAIMER

With this book I hope to enhance our current knowledge of health and our health care system by focusing on each patient's responsibility to take control of his or her health by understanding the concept of, and exercising the right to, informed consent. However, nothing in this book should be interpreted as a suggestion to readers to dismiss the advice of any other health care provider.

I hope that by providing a simple step-by-step method to achieving better health I can help readers reduce their risk of developing some of the most devastating chronic degenerative diseases of our time, and teach their children to do the same. If readers were to follow these basic steps I believe we, as a society, could reduce suffering at a population level, focus the remarkable advances made by allopathic medicine on those for whom prevention is not enough, and make health care more affordable for all of us. However, direct consultation with a qualified health care provider will always be better than general comments written for a broad audience.

INTRODUCTION

"The doctor of the future will give no medicine but will interest his patients in the care of the human frame, in a proper diet, and in the cause and prevention of disease."

THOMAS A. EDISON
(1847 - 1931)

Hello, I am Dr. Raj Jheeta, ND, and I believe the Doctor of the Future is here.

Let me explain: to start let's take a closer look at the first part of Thomas Edison's quotation, where he says, "the doctor of the future will give no medicine..." This idea is very encouraging, after all the possibility of not having to take medication is something that appeals to almost everyone. But, you might be thinking since so much time has passed since the early 1900's, that by now Mr. Edison would expect the Doctor of the Future to actually have some kind of high-tech Star Trek-like device to diagnose and treat his patients with – but unfortunately, we all know that technology does not yet exist.

As you read the last part of the quotation perhaps we get a better idea of what he really meant: "...but (he the doctor) will interest (educate) his patients in the care of the human frame, in a proper diet, and in the cause and prevention of disease." So now we understand what he is really pointing out, that the Doctor of the Future will educate his patients about their bodies', a proper diet and the concept of true prevention with the ultimate goal of reducing the risk of developing chronic degenerative diseases such as diabetes, heart disease, arthritis, autoimmune disease, and even some cancers. This is something I believe is possible. The only question remaining in my mind is, until everyone has received a higher level of health education, what can we do in the mean time?

This is where I believe I have an answer.

The Doctor of the Future I am referring to understands first and foremost the importance of educating the patient because most of the time an educated patient eventually becomes a healthy patient! The Doctor of the Future also has a number of other important attributes that aid him in this quest to educate his patients:

1. **Is a highly trained and licensed professional in preventative medicine**
2. **Believes that education is the key to true prevention**
3. **Applies an integrated approach to healing, and**
4. **Believes everyone should invest time and money into health education**

The most comforting thing for you to know is that these types of doctors exist today. As a matter of fact I am one of them, and I do all of these things daily, and so do many of my associates. I am a licensed professional who focuses on prevention by using diagnostic tools to assess the patient's level of health, not their level of sickness – this is called a naturopathic approach. I also use traditional diagnosis to determine the cause of a disease and may also recommend prescription drugs to eliminate the signs and symptoms of a disease, this is called an allopathic approach. The objective in all cases is to find the right treatment options that will support and improve the body's healing potential. Above all, I aim to educate my patients so they can help prevent the recurrence of their own health issues.

Years ago, I began creating teaching tools for young professional doctors to help them communicate this important message of prevention and accountability in order to remedy this situation. However, I soon realized I hadn't gone far enough, as I now believe everyone needs to learn how to take back control of their health. This is why I wrote this book and simplified the tools I created, so you too can understand that there are many things you can do to prevent disease and stay healthy. These tools, the 3P's, Generational Health First, Dr. Jheeta's Algorithm, and the Three E's, will give you health knowledge that most people have never had before.

Don't be a "WILLING VICTIM" and have no choice other than to manage a diseased state with necessary yet potentially dangerous drugs.

Thomas Edison's quotation is a source of inspiration guiding us to make health education a priority for everyone – so that each and every person can learn how to take back control of their own health.

HOW I ARRIVED AT MY DESTINATION

In 1983, I made a decision that has shaped my life ever since: I decided to become a naturopathic doctor (ND). Having studied biology and botany at the University of British Columbia, I was interested in both the growing environmental movement and the potential for botanical medicine to promote health. In the 80's naturopathy was a young profession and when I graduated in 1987, I was the fifty-third registered naturopathic doctor in Canada; nevertheless, I saw it as the way of the future and I wanted to be part of it.

Looking back, I confess, that as a budding doctor, I was cocky, at least with regard to my views on health. I started my naturopathic education with some very one-sided, negative beliefs about allopathic (traditional) health care and its ties with the pharmaceutical industry. I felt there was no place at all for drugs in health care and that allopathic medicine should be used only in case of acute trauma or immediately life-threatening illness. Then again, I was 22 years old and in great health.

At the college, we often worked in teams with real patients. In one case, a young man came to us with severe migraines and a bag full of medicines ranging from routine analgesics, like Tylenol, to opiates, which are powerful, addictive drugs. The drugs were having terrible impacts on his life. He couldn't hold down a job because he couldn't stay alert, he was constantly nauseated, and he had dramatic mood swings. His allopathic doctors had made no effort to identify the source of his headaches. They'd said his only choice was to cycle through the drugs until he found the right combination, and then continue using them for the rest of his life. He wasn't prepared to accept that.

Our team began to investigate possible causes of his headaches. We evaluated his musculoskeletal system, food sensitivities, stress levels, sleep patterns, and hydration. We recommended minerals to relieve muscle tension, and herbal supplements to improve his circulation. Gradually, he found that his pain medication was working more quickly and effectively, and thus he reduced his dosage. Slowly, the frequency of his headaches decreased from daily to weekly to once every few months. Eventually, the severity lessened so much that he was able to use only over-the-counter (OTC) painkillers to relieve his pain. Our success with him and others like him bolstered our belief that we were on the one and only right path to health.

THE MEDICAL CASTLE ON PILL HILL

When I was in university, there was only one naturopathic college in North America and it was located in a converted elementary school in a suburb of Portland, Oregon. Portland's Medical Science Institute for allopathic medicine was situated across town, on the other side of the bridge, up on the hill, in a wealthy area on the west side of the city. We called it "Pill Hill." The whole situation had a fairy-tale-like quality to it, as if dragons might fly out the windows of the medical school and, in one fiery breath, raze our poor little college to the ground. We were David. They were Goliath!

Once in a while, representatives of the medical school would visit us. Perhaps they were checking out the competition, looking for reasons to put us out of business. Our college was in the process of accreditation, which we needed to secure student loans and other funding. We knew all too well that a wrong word from the visitors of "Pill Hill" could jeopardize all our hopes and dreams. Yet, in what I see now as arrogance on our part, we believed, in black and white terms, that the patients, like the young man with migraines, demonstrated how allopathic care was bad and naturopathic care was good. So in spite of our fears, during those visits we made no secret of our crusade to expose what we saw as allopathic medicine's real agenda; an agenda we thought had more to do with corporate wealth than patient wellness.

We saw those visitors as ignorant, prejudiced, and perhaps even fearful of our new paradigm of health. Our philosophies were polar opposites. Hostility was constant. We made no effort to find common ground. In hindsight, I can now see two things clearly that I could not see before: first, our visitors' ignorance, prejudice, and fear was in no small measure our own fault and second, it was also a mirror reflecting our own ignorance, prejudice, and fear of them right back at us.

NATUROPATHY'S FIGHT TO SURVIVE

Sometimes, some of the naturopathic students would embark on "field trips" across the bridge to the allopathic medical school in the upscale part of town. We'd hang out there and get into heated debates with the students, arguing about whether to suppress or support a fever, mask pain with drugs or use it to seek underlying causes. Whatever the topic, the debates were always marked by a very us-and-them feel. The term integrated care was not yet in anyone's vocabulary.

I remember one debate clearly: it was about antibiotics. We explained our philosophy that every living thing has a life force and will adapt to its environment to survive. We expressed concern that overuse of antibiotics would cause bacteria to evolve to a point where they would be so powerful no drug could kill them. The allopathic students thought it was ridiculous to think single-celled creatures could have a life force. They shared their opinions of our theories, and their thoughts about us, in no uncertain terms. Our words grew hostile, our voices loud, and our posturing aggressive. In the end, fearing someone might call campus security to escort us from the building, my classmates and I left and made our way back down the hill and across the bridge, to our converted elementary school in the suburbs.

In some ways, it's amazing naturopathy survived. We were always under threat of a sunset law, which meant if naturopathic medicine did not prove itself worthy within a certain period of time, it would cease to exist as a recognized discipline. On one side, there was intense lobbying from powerful people to abolish naturopathic medicine in Oregon. On the other side, we'd successfully treated enough patients that our supporters circulated petitions and gathered enough signatures that state politicians (likely more concerned about re-election than informed about naturopathy) let us continue to exist.

A SHIFT IN MY PERSPECTIVE

I remained dogmatic in my opinions, as did most of my classmates, until my fourth and final year, when we were working as externs (similar to an intern, but an extern may work either within the college or in an NDs' private practice). We took turns leading teams and, by that time, I'd been the primary clinician on several routine cases. Usually, we'd examine the patient, consult as a team, formulate a treatment protocol, and send the patient home with remedies and instructions, and that would be that.

Occasionally, we'd have a patient who was in significant pain, but we would never veer from our principle of prevention rather than palliation. Naturopathic doctors believe the path to health lies in discovering what's causing symptoms and preventing those underlying causes from developing into diseases. This is very different from the allopathic approach of waiting until diseases have developed and can be diagnosed, and then using palliative measures, like painkillers, to treat symptoms without addressing underlying causes.

Even when we had a patient who was in considerable pain, we believed providing painkillers would only make it more difficult to identify and treat underlying causes, and might also complicate the patient's problems with adverse drug effects. We recommended natural pain remedies (which are rarely as effective as drugs), sent the patient home knowing he was still in pain, and then slept comfortably because we felt we were serving the greater good.

Then we had a case that changed my perspective. The patient was a pleasant Latina woman in her thirties. She and her husband had three young children. Their family was immersed in the naturopathic approach to living. There was just one large problem:

she had stage 4 cervical cancer. Our treatment protocol for this was a vag pac, a concoction of herbs with properties toxic to cancer cells. Applied externally, it was designed to do the same thing as the drugs, but it worked much more slowly. It might have been appropriate at an earlier stage, but she didn't have that much time. If a naturopathic doctor were to use a vag pac on stage 4 cancer today, her license to practice would be revoked.

Beyond the urgency of her disease, this woman was also in severe pain. I encouraged her to pursue relief through whatever means necessary. In fact, I urged her to go to an allopathic doctor for surgery and drug treatment for the cancer, as well as palliative care for the pain, but she and her husband were steadfast in their beliefs in naturopathic medicine. I remain certain, even now, that if she'd accepted allopathic treatment, she might still be alive today. Instead, her children grew up without their mother.

In some ways, I have to thank that woman. Tragically, she showed me that my course as a new doctor must be to advocate an integrated approach to health care. It became clear to me that it had never been a case of us versus the or naturopathic medicine versus allopathic medicine. Though my classmates began to see me as a bit of a weak link, I began to realize that we had gotten it all wrong. The real skill was not to learn one approach and stick to it rigidly, but to understand both approaches and know when and how it was appropriate to implement each of them.

Private Practice and The 3Ps

I was fortunate enough to start my own private practice in 1988. At the time, a friend of my brother's happened to be studying allopathic medicine, which was a fortunate turn of events for both of us, as it gave us both someone to talk to and debate with. It wasn't like those debates on Pill Hill. I'd known him for a long time and we respected each other. Because of this, and also because of that experience in fourth year, I listened to his stories and agreed that sometimes drugs were necessary. At the same time, because of the examples he was seeing every day, of drugs being overused and patients suffering, he also agreed that drugs were not always the answer.

Over the next several years, the idea of the 3 Ps began to take shape in my mind. The 3 Ps is my shorthand for profits, products, and people. It's a concept I came up with for thinking about how our culture and our health system today evolved out of the Industrial Revolution. Yes, you read that correctly, and I'll explain what I mean in Chapter 1.

The important thing here is that my concept of the 3 Ps became a way for me to understand corporate decision-making, and to see that in real life there are no fairy-tale kings, dragons, or villagers. The 3 Ps simply represent a way of doing business. It's not all good and it's not all bad. Like most things in life, it's both, and each of us has to learn to understand it well enough to make it work for us in our own lives.

Whenever I'm tempted to blame corporations for the health issues I see in my patients every day, the 3 Ps remind me that corporations are not to blame. They're doing what they're supposed to do, which is make a profit. That's what they're accountable to their shareholders for doing. They're not responsible for our health. WE ARE! Each of us, as individuals. It's our job to recognize the risk factors for illness and work proactively to prevent it, not wait until we're sick and then take reactive measures.

We're all responsible for every health decision we make, from the kind of food we eat to the treatments we consent to. But we can only take responsibility by learning enough to provide *informed consent.* We can't rely on doctors or corporations to tell us what to do, and we can't blame them when information was available to us yet we still made poor choices. Sometimes, the consequences of ignoring information and making poor health choices can be minor, but other times they can be devastating. That's why each of us needs to be more accountable for our own health and teach our children to do the same, now, before it's too late.

FIGHTING DISEASES OF AFFLUENCE

One of the most significant things to come from the Industrial Revolution was a shift from the collective responsibility that is common in traditional and often pre-industrial cultures to the individual responsibility that forms the basis for most industrial societies. Good or bad, right or wrong, we are now living with the full impacts of the Industrial Revolution on our culture, environment, food, and health.

There have been many consequences of the Industrial Revolution and we haven't fully adapted to them yet. For example, corporations that are responsible primarily for making profits have invented or developed products that earn them profit because people enjoy them enough to buy them, but they are not necessarily good for people's health.

We see this in products like foods made with refined sugar and processed fats, foods we've discovered over the past 25 years are not just benign pleasures but are actually both addictive and, when used to excess over the long term, can even be lethal. We are now experiencing the results of excessive, long-term use of these products in the development of chronic degenerative conditions like heart disease, diabetes, cancer, and arthritis.

Cardiovascular and cerebrovascular diseases (CVD),[†] diabetes, and hypertension are some of the biggest killers in Canada and America today, but they are considered diseases of affluence. According to the World Health Organization (WHO), in lower-income nations, people are most likely to die of communicable diseases that cause respiratory illness such as AIDS or diarrhea.

But in high-income nations like Canada and the US, people are most likely to die of non-communicable diseases that arise from a combination of too little physical activity and too much consumption. At the root of these differences is lifestyle: a growing trend in the decades since World War II toward increasingly stressful but sedentary lives, combined with diets high in refined carbohydrates, processed fats, and salt, and not enough unrefined foods or exercise.

This trend has been become increasingly clear for decades, and statistics from the World Health Organization (WHO) for deaths in North and South America (all ages, both sexes) suggest that it's not going to change any time soon:

- In 2000, when a total of 5.5 million people died in North and South America combined, about 4.2 million died of non-communicable diseases (NCD's), chiefly CVD, various cancers, and diabetes.

---

† CVD refers to various forms of heart disease and stroke.

- In 2011, when a total of 6.3 million people died in North and South America, about 5 million died of NCDs, chiefly CVD, various cancers, and diabetes.
- In 2015, the WHO projects that 6.6 million people will die in North and South America, and about 5.3 million will die of NCDs, chiefly CVD, various cancers, and diabetes.
- In 2030, the WHO projects that 8.6 million people will die in North and South America, and about 7.1 million will die of NCDs, chiefly CVD, various cancers, and diabetes.

Do you see the trend toward an increasing number of people dying of these devastating yet completely preventable diseases? I'll talk more about this throughout Part I. For now, the most important point is that, while it's tempting to blame corporations for selling us products that made us sick, ultimately the responsibility is not theirs. Their primary responsibility is to be profitable. Our health is our own responsibility. It's up to each of us to make intelligent, informed decisions.

PUTTING GENERATIONAL HEALTH FIRST

Over the early years of my private practice, as my understanding of the 3 Ps began to take shape in my mind, so did another concept, the idea of putting your health first, and passing that knowledge on to your children, or what I call Generational Health First. At it's simplest; Generational Health First is about habits - good habits and bad habits - and what we choose to do with them.

Habits are hard to break. This is equally true whether they're good habits or bad ones. If you don't believe me, try going without brushing your teeth for the next month. I bet you wouldn't last a week! That's because your parents made a healthy choice to have you brush your teeth every day, and they taught you that choice when you were so young it became second nature to you.

Over nearly 30 years of private practice, I've seen Generational Health First in action many times. Parents take the difficult step of changing bad health habits into good ones, and then they teach those good health habits to their children, and their children grow up practicing those healthy habits as if they were second nature.

Generational Health First is a term I coined. It's not yet a term that's on everyone's lip, but I hope it will be soon. And then I hope it won't be. I hope it will be, because I think that's what it will take for people to begin thinking about their health as a responsibility they have to themselves, and to others.

And then I hope it won't be, because it will become so common no one will need to say it anymore. By the time our great-grandchildren are born, I hope they won't be talking about putting Generational Health First. I hope they won't have to, because it will be second nature to them.

DR. JHEETA'S ALGORITHM

It all sounds very idealistic, but the puzzle to me has always been how to get there from here. Then, several years ago, I realized we were already on our way. I began noticing more NDs moving toward integrating allopathic and naturopathic medicine, toward recognizing that, where one didn't work, the other might, and sometimes they worked best together. I also began noticing some MDs were catching on to this idea.

That's when I began thinking about the doctor of the future. I realized that, if the idea of putting Generational Health First took hold, both allopathic and naturopathic doctors would have to adapt. The doctor of the future would integrate allopathic and naturopathic care, and that was when I began formulating Dr. Jheeta's Algorithm, a system to educate young naturopathic doctors about what I have learned over the decades in my practise. Then, after further contemplation about what the future of health care might look like, I came to the conclusion that everyone must have this knowledge. This is why I simplified the explanation of the processes in my algorithm, so that everyone not just professionals, could learn how to take back control of their health. Dr. Jheeta's Algorithm is the centerpiece of this book, both literally and figuratively (see Figure 1 on page 112). It's the smallest part of the book, but can be the most powerful.

THE THREE E'S

The Three E's, Education, Evaluation and Empowerment, is a concept I created that works not only for the purposes of health and this book, but can also be applied in your everyday life. For example: When buying a house for the first time, it's one of the largest purchases you will ever make in your life and could easily affect your finances for many years to come. So before buying what do you do? Do you research the housing market, do you learn about features and attributes you require, do you take advise from a professional in that market? Of course you do, you educate yourself before you buy. Buying at the wrong time or in the wrong location could cost you thousands of dollars. So research, investigation, and historical evidence are all part of the process of educating yourself. How can you make an informed decision without it?

Before you buy a home do you do an inspection to discover whether it needs a new roof or if the pipes need to be replaced? Of course you do. You want to assess what the condition of the house is before you can make an informed decision on whether to buy it. To do a proper assessment or evaluation, you either have to hire a professional who will explain what condition the house is in, this is where you learn about what parameters are involved in making this type of assessment. Or you may already have many years of experience looking inside houses and understand how they are built and what factors are necessary for a final assessment.

Regardless of your experience level, type of purchase you are making or type of decision that is being made. The more education you have and the more experience you have in doing an evaluation will both empower you to make a more informed decision. I believe the Three E's is the lens through which you should view how your body works and how to make the right health decisions from this day forward. I hope to show you that the doctor of the future is really a conduit that provides knowledge, using my Three E's approach to health: Part I: Education, provides the background for understanding the health industry today, Part II: Evaluation, how to use Dr. Jheeta's Algorithm, Part III: Empowerment, shows you how to use education and proper evaluation to empower yourself to take back control of your health.

Here's a slightly different way of looking at the way the book is laid out:

- Part I: Education: how our health issues and health-care system evolved into what they are today
- Part II: Evaluation: what I actually do in my clinical practice to address patients' health care issues
- Part III: Empowerment: what you can do to address your health care issues on your own and together with a health care professional

PART I: EDUCATION

INTRODUCTION TO INFORMED CONSENT

A century ago, before health insurance was available, and before a lot of changes took place in our environment and food supply, people had to take control of their own health, since there was no national health care system back then. They couldn't afford to run to the doctor every time their child had a sniffle, so they did things like insisting their children take a spoonful of cod liver oil daily.

A century ago, people were not as well educated and informed about health as we are today – or as we could be. Mothers today feed their children cod liver oil because they learned on the internet that it's rich in essential fatty acids (EFA) that bolster the immune system. They also do it because they learned it from their mothers and grandmothers.

A century ago, people practised preventative health care by eating healthy food and getting plenty of exercise, but they typically didn't think it as having a healthy lifestyle, they just thought of it as living.

A century ago, when people went to the doctor, it was usually because someone had been in an accident or was seriously ill. Patients were unlikely to question their doctor's advice, and if they did, the doctor was likely to respond with, "When did you become an MD?" Meaning, "How dare you question me!"

That unquestioning attitude has carried over into this century, even though the situation today is very different. We go to the doctor much more often and for much lesser concerns than people did a century ago, and we have many more treatment options. Each of those treatments carries risks and benefits, and we have knowledge to help us weigh those risks and benefits, but few of us understand how to do that.

This is the challenge. Having knowledge about treatment options, asking questions, and expecting answers are crucial to the principle of informed consent, which, in turn, is crucial to the practice of medicine, whether naturopathic or allopathic. However, most patients don't really understand what it means or that it refers to researching risks and benefits, above and beyond what your doctor tells you, and then making the choices you've decided are right for you on the basis of the information you've found.

Informed consent must start with education. That's why Part I of this book provides an educational background to help you understand that our culture has lost control of the health care system, and that perhaps you, in your life, have also lost control of your health. I will not pretend that the background information I provide in Part I is complete. It's only a starting point. It's intended to inspire you to seek more information.

I also won't pretend it's unbiased. I have clearly stated my beliefs in the Introduction, and I will continue to expand upon them throughout the book. Whenever an expert provides you with information, you need to take their bias into account. No matter how hard any health professional tries to be objective, they will always have a bias.

It's important for you to understand their bias, and seek information to balance it. When you read this book, you need to take my bias into account, too. Having information and understanding different experts' biases are the only ways to ensure that when, the time comes for you to consider any kind of health treatment, whether it's a prescription for antibiotics or a recommendation for major surgery, you are able to provide informed consent.

Chapter 1: health: how do we learn from the past?

What does the Industrial Revolution have to do with the evolution of your health? I understand why you might think it's an odd connection. So let me start this chapter, as I will start most of them, with a story.

In her grade 10 year, the daughter of a friend started having abdominal pain. It grew worse and worse all year until finally my friend decided to homeschool her daughter for the last two months of the school year. She did this as part of a two-pronged, naturopathic and allopathic offensive against the pain. My friend has long believed in integrated health care and, given some of her own medical history, she wasn't taking any chances with her daughter's health.

"I was worried," my friend said. "I thought my daughter's problems were stress-related, but I have Crohn's disease, which has a strong genetic component (another family member also has it). It was possible my daughter could be in the early stages of Crohn's, so I took allopathic precautions. But I didn't want to rule out anything else, so I also took her to our naturopathic doctor."

My friend booked an appointment to have her daughter allopathically tested for the characteristic ulceration caused by Crohn's, but there was a wait of several months. In the meantime, they followed the ND's advice. At the same time, she spent every weekday morning sitting at the kitchen table, trying to help her daughter understand the Industrial Revolution, unsure why she was finding this important bit of history so difficult to digest.

"It's confusing and irrelevant," her daughter often said. "What does it have to do with me?"

"Well, I can't say just yet," her mother told her. "But, it's usually good to learn about history. Maybe you should just believe that your parents and teachers aren't trying to torture you, and have faith that someday, something will happen in your life, and it will suddenly become clear: this was why I had to learn about the Industrial Revolution."

Somehow, mother and daughter made it through the school year and when the daughter wrote her year-end social studies exam, she passed with flying colours.

Over the summer, she laid low and nursed her nagging but slowly lessening abdominal pain. When fall came, she decided she'd rather be at school with her friends than lying around at home, even when her gut hurt. It wasn't until a year later, my friend said, (after they'd ruled out Crohn's disease) that they found out what the real problem was.

"My daughter was diagnosed with a reading disability," she said. "She was in grade 11, but still reading at a grade 9 level. She'd been struggling to keep up with her peers at school since grade 9.Yet none of her teachers or allopathic doctors had thought to go deeper to find the root causes of her abdominal pain," she said.

The teachers had written off her falling grades as "not trying hard enough," while the doctors had said there was nothing organic wrong, implying that the teachers were right.

"I'd continued to wonder if it was stress," she said. "The ND had treated her for stress. Between the naturopathic treatment and getting help with reading the book on the Industrial Revolution, which she was probably having trouble with because of her learning disability, she'd been able to go back to school. But it was only when the school paid real attention to the underlying problem and helped with her reading disability that her stress issues were finally resolved."

My friend's daughter recently completed her B.A. and embarked on a career she's thrilled about. So, even if the Industrial Revolution never means anything else to her, it will always remind her that where there's pain, there's an explanation, and it's not always the explanation that meets the eye.

THE 3 PS

You don't need a learning disability to think the details of the Industrial Revolution are little more than a pain in your gut. In high school, I too wondered why I needed to learn about this, but in the early years of my practice, I found myself thinking about it often and how it might relate to health in modern times.

Eventually, I came up with a concept I call the 3 Ps, which stands for profit, product, and people. This concept has often helped me understand the many contradictions I've struggled with, such as how pharmaceuticals can sometimes be life saving while other times they make patients even sicker. In my practice today, I often use the 3 Ps to help patients understand the roles they play in their own sickness and health, not to blame them, but to encourage them to take responsibility for their health.

Hippocrates said, "let food be thy medicine and medicine be thy food." What he meant was, if you're ill, the right food can help you get well, and if you're well, the right food can help you avoid illness.

What does Hippocrates have to do with the Industrial Revolution or the 3 Ps?

A lot. But in case you don't remember what you learned about it in high school, let me refresh your memory.

The Industrial Revolution was a period of time when a rapid series of changes in manufacturing processes dramatically altered our way of life. The Industrial Revolution, and much of what we take for granted about life today, would not have been possible if not for the Agricultural Revolution, which began about a century earlier (around 1600) and continued alongside the Industrial Revolution (about 1700 to 1850).

The Agricultural Revolution began with inventions like the Dutch plough, the seed driller, and four-crop rotation. With these methods, tilling fields became less labour-intensive, seed germination became more certain, and farmers were able to plant all their fields every year rather than letting some fields lie fallow (grow wild) for a year or two to restore soil nutrients depleted by previous crops.

Another change during the Agricultural Revolution was that landowners won the right to build fences around their land. Until then, a few people owned land but whole villages shared the work and the harvest, with a little left over for the landowner's profit. As new inventions made farming more profitable, landowners built fences to keep people out – the same people who had previously helped them work their land. So wealthy landowners became wealthier, and poor families fled to the cities looking for work.

By this time, the Industrial Revolution was in full swing in the cities. New machinery had sped up the process of spinning cotton and wool into thread and knitting or weaving it into fabric. Textile factories dotted the cityscape, their chimneys blackening the sky with thick smoke from coal furnaces. Displaced farm families trickled, and then streamed, and then poured, into the cities, resulting in large crowds and unsanitary housing that was often infested with rats and infected with disease.

In other words, a wealthy few enjoyed tremendous profits generated by the sale of mass-produced products, but their wealth came at the expense of poorer people. Hence, the 3 Ps: profits first, products second, people third. Profits, products, people. This simple phrase has helped me understand, and has helped hundreds of my patients understand, how our health care system works, what their role in it is, and why it's important for them to take responsibility for their own health.

NO CONSPIRACY THEORIES

I want to be very clear: I don't believe in conspiracy theories. That's not what the 3 Ps are about. I don't think it does any good to blame the system or anyone who's playing their role in it for anything bad that happens. I don't judge whether the Industrial Revolution was good or bad. It was both.

What was good about it?

It gave rise to our way of life, and there's a lot of good in our way of life. For example, when a lot of wealth is concentrated in a few hands, it allows for advances in technology, science, art, education, sports, and medicine that would not otherwise be possible. From lights that brighten our homes to cell phones that keep us in touch to over-the-counter painkillers and cancer-killing chemotherapies, it's hard to name anything about our way of life today that can't be traced back to the Industrial Revolution.

What about the bad side?

I'll get back to that. First, I want to talk a little more about the Agricultural Revolution. Actually, it's wrong to call it the Agricultural Revolution, because there have been at least three. The first one happened 10,000 years ago when hunting-and-gathering cultures realized they could settle down in one spot and grow crops. The second one (the one I've been talking about) changed farming from a subsistence activity (growing enough to feed your family) to mass production of food for considerable profit. The third one occurred in the last century, mostly since World War II, and took mass production of food to a whole new level.

THE THIRD REVOLUTION

Although the idea of the 3 Ps came to me when I was thinking about the Industrial Revolution, it's the most recent agricultural revolution that reminds me most of what Hippocrates said about letting food be our medicine. The third agricultural revolution raises new questions about the 3 Ps, and how mass-producing food relates to our health and health care system today.

Before World War II, one-third to one-half of Canadians and Americans lived on farms and grew food for the rest of us. If a customer didn't like the quality of your roast beef or if his milk went sour too quickly, he could chat directly with farmer Joe at the general store when he came into town for supplies, or when the two of them were tossing horseshoes after church on Sunday. The farmer, in those days, was directly accountable to his customers for the quality of food he produced; the people he served had to be his highest priority, or he wouldn't make money.

After the war, everything changed. One of the first changes was in the population. As soldiers came home and got married, the population boomed – that's right, the baby boomers – while at the same time sons and daughters of many farm families moved to the city looking for better lives. A growing number of people needed food, but there were fewer farmers to feed them. Fortunately, even before the war, advances in agricultural knowledge and technology were making it possible to grow more crops on the same amount of land.

23

But the advances weren't only about growing more food to feed the booming population at home. International markets were opening up, economic prosperity was growing, and agriculture was the backbone of that prosperity. Government and industry quickly saw investments in agriculture as business opportunities that would help grow both private companies and national economies. Some researchers developed chemical fertilizers that made crop rotation a thing of the past, and others developed seeds with pest-resistant properties, while engineers designed and built larger and larger equipment to do the work.

The ingenuity was astounding – and expensive. Over the decades, many farmers who tried to keep up with the advances became mired in debt, declared bankruptcy, and had to quit farming. Large companies bought the land and consolidated many small farms into fewer but larger farms. They then used these large farms to increase their profits and finance more technological advances.

Are you talking about the bad side now?

Yes. In some cases, farm families faced the devastating possibility of losing land, and a way of life, that had been in their families for generations. To avoid this, some farmers signed contracts with growing multinational food corporations. In fact, many farms today operate under such contracts. I'll talk about that more in Chapter 2.

The main point is that corporations buy farmers' goods and sell them under their brand name. Customers buy those products because they recognize and trust the brand. Corporations then provide farm families with steady income, and allow them to stay on their land and continue a way of life most of them wouldn't trade for all the wealth in the world.

In return, however, corporations require farmers to grow their products according to the exact specifications customers expect of that brand. Sometimes, contracts between corporations and farmers require farmers to buy fertilizers, equipment, and much more from specific, affiliated agribusiness corporations. The promise to farmers is a kind of security that's rare in farming, while the promise to customers is a product that's always the same.

WE DON'T KNOW

In some ways, it seems like an ideal system. But when I started really thinking about it many years ago, it raised a lot of questions for me, questions like:

- What does it mean for our health when food is produced in more and more massive quantities by fewer and fewer farmers for greater and greater profits?
- What does it mean for our health when farmers are forced to use chemical fertilizers, hybridized seeds, and other products even if they don't believe that's the best way to grow healthy food?
- What does it mean for our health when farms are not run by people, but huge agribusinesses whose priorities are: first, profits for shareholders, second, products that will generate those profits, and only third, the health of the people eating the food?

What are the answers?

I don't have all the answers, but I do know the economic system that emerged from the Industrial Revolution doesn't put people first, the way farmer Joe did. I know that if profits are the highest priority, agribusinesses and food corporations probably aren't thinking about Hippocrates, because his idea about food as medicine might be good for people, but probably not for profits.

Okay, but isn't that where organically grown food comes in? Aren't more and more farmers growing organic? Can't people just choose organic if they want healthier food?

That's one option, although, it may not be a realistic one for everyone. Often organic can be cost prohibitive for families on a budget and it can be difficult to find organic produce in poorer neighbourhoods around North America. Another issue that needs to be addressed here is the question of whether organically grown food is actually more nutritious than mass-produced foods.

That seems like it should be a no-brainer!

It does, but it's not. A blog post for *Scientific American,* written by an author who seems to favour organic foods theoretically, summed up the whole issue this way:

Sorry to say, but as of now, there is no clear-cut answer as to whether organic foods are nutritionally advanced as compared to conventionally grown foods. Several studies have reported an increase in vitamin, mineral, and phytochemical content of organic produce, and while I would LOVE to believe them, these findings must be taken with a grain of salt due to the major problems with study design variability and just poor science in some cases. Not only do we need more quality studies looking into this question, we need more studies examining the bioavailability [form of the nutrients that may make nutritional content easier or harder for the body to absorb] of organic vs. conventional foods . . .

[However,] I'm just talking nutrients here—whether fertilizers and pesticides used in conventional farming methods have health effects is [another] issue . . . [*]

This raises two issues that fit with a naturopathic view of health. First, the studies saying there's no difference in nutritional content aren't looking at bioavailability, which is important in naturopathy, while studies saying there is a difference – don't comply with rigorous scientific standards.

Is this a 3 Ps issue – like who funds which studies, and therefore how well they're done?

It could be, and I hope someone with the right qualifications and good funding will follow up on that. But the second point, the one the author tacks on about fertilizers and pesticides almost as an afterthought, is more interesting to me.

Why?

Because even though companies say these chemicals have no negative health effects, they provide suggestions for making the produce grown with them safer. That in itself is puzzling, but their suggestions for making it safer are even more puzzling. For example:

---

[*] "Nutritional Differences in Organic versus Conventional Foods: And the Winner Is..." by Erin Prosser, August 11, 2011, *Scientific American* blog, http://blogs.scientificamerican.com/guest-blog/2011/08/11/nutritional-differences-in-organic-vs-conventional-foods-and-the-winner-is/.

- They suggest washing produce well, but pesticides don't just sit on the surface of the produce, they penetrate it, so washing won't completely get rid of them.
- They suggest peeling the produce, but that does reduce nutritional content, because nutrients are most concentrated in the skin.
- They don't suggest anything to compensate for mass-produced food often being shipped from very far away, which means it was picked before it was ripe, which also reduces nutritional value.
- They suggest eating a varied diet so we don't ingest too much of any one pesticide, but why would we think it's better to ingest small amounts of several pesticides than large amounts of one or two?

My point is that it's all very contradictory, and the contradictions don't only make it difficult to accept these suggestions at face value, they also make it difficult to accept research saying there is no nutritional difference between organic and mass-produced. But for now, just keep that in mind.

TAKING RESPONSIBILITY

When you think about mass-produced food with the 3 Ps in mind – not to get into blame or conspiracy theories, just to understand that large corporations put profits first because that's the way they become large – you have to ask yourself whether you want to continue eating mass-produced food. Is the money you save worth risks to your health that we just don't know about yet?

If it is, that's fine, because my goal is not for you to do what I tell you to do, my goal is for you to take responsibility for your health. If you gather information, think it through, and make a decision, you're taking responsibility. However, before you decide you may want to read the next chapter to better understand the connections between mass agricultural production and the well-known impacts of the fast food industry on our health today.

CHAPTER 2:
HOW – AND WHY – DID FOOD BECOME FAST?

In the early 1960s, my parents bought our first television. Suddenly, we could see people all across the country living just like us. I remember the soap operas that became wildly popular during the 1960s and 1970s. The characters were like our neighbours, except they were living dramatic and riveting lives. They lived in nice homes and wore fabulous clothes, and we all wanted what they had.

That was the point. Those shows were called "soap operas" because at first they were sponsored by soap companies to engage housewives' undivided attention during the day time and advertise products to them. It was an ingenious technique that became more effective as the price of TVs came down. Corporations could create demand, not just for products, but for a whole lifestyle.

As demand grew for the increasingly extravagant lives depicted on TV, more families needed two incomes to keep up. That created a demand for fast-cooking foods that could be put on the table after both parents came home from a long day of work, or meals that kids could make for themselves in their parents' absence.

"Let me know when the Kraft Dinner commercial comes on," my mother would say from the kitchen.

"Mom, you do know it's backward to skip the show and watch the commercials, right?"

"Not for me," she'd say. "I want to see the next step in tonight's Kraft Dinner recipe."

We wouldn't argue or tease anymore because we wanted her to learn how to make those meals, too. They were quick, easy, affordable, and delicious. We were hooked!

It was not until many years later that I began to understand how a box of white pasta and powdered cheese could contribute to the epidemic of chronic degenerative diseases, which in many instances could have been avoided by eating healthy, unprocessed foods in the first place.

CONVENIENT AND PROFITABLE

It's tempting to say convenience food had its start in the 1950s, 1960s, and 1970s, but it, too, originated during the Industrial Revolution. The first canned foods, primarily meats, were created during the Napoleonic Wars (1803–1815) to feed troops in the field. Over the next century, the cost of canning lessened, and during the Victorian era, it became customary to keep canned foods on the shelf to avoid the need to go to the market every day. Canned goods were really the first convenience foods.

During World War I and II, increasing demand for high-calorie "rations" that troops could transport in their backpacks led to the development of frozen and freeze-dried foods. After World War II, food companies that had invested time and money developing these products began marketing them to housewives as convenience foods. Food and chemical companies developed new methods of food processing to give food longer shelf lives. The burgeoning advertising industry used the growing popularity of television to persuade housewives that freeze-dried mashed potatoes and five-minute rice were the answers to their busy lives.

Food companies marketed processed foods, ranging from vegetable margarines to powdered fruit juice, cake mixes, and white bread, as featuring numerous benefits. For example, foods that had been precooked were quick and convenient for families on the go. Foods that had been processed to extend shelf life protected families from the cost and potential illness of spoilage. White bread appealed to children who were picky eaters and had so many vitamins and minerals added that one brand was called "Wonder Bread." Margarine made from hydrogenated vegetable oil stayed soft and spreadable in the refrigerator, and tasted "just like butter" but was supposed to be better for health. Powdered orange juice was less expensive than fresh squeezed – and if NASA astronauts drank it in space, it must be good!

But the truth had little to do with benefits to customers; processing foods and adding preservatives reduced spoilage during shipping or in the store, and increased profits. Food corporations developed, tested, and marketed new products with amazing frequency, growing in size and wealth in the process.

The food processing companies were not the only ones to profit: so did the agribusinesses that grew the foods, the chemical companies that developed the artificial flavours, colours, and preservatives, the supermarket chains that used popular brands to lure customers, the shipping companies that transported everything from one end of the country to the other, the engineering companies that designed production equipment, the construction companies that built processing plants and grocery stores, and the advertising companies that developed massive marketing campaigns – the list goes on and on. Mass production and overconsumption were the twin engines driving the prosperity everyone enjoyed.

NOT A SINGLE STRAWBERRY

There's actually nothing new about fast food. Street vendors have sold meat pies, fish and chips, pizza, kebabs, and the like for centuries. But what we think of as fast food today – burgers, fries, and shakes – got its start just after World War I.

Howard Johnson's and A&W opened the first drive-ins, focusing on a small menu, fast service, high volumes, and low prices. McDonald's started out as a drive-in, but in 1948 they put up their golden arches and converted to the walk-in, assembly-line restaurant we know today. TV commercials seduced viewers with images of happy families eating delicious, affordable food in casual restaurants, and soon fast-food joints included Dunkin' Donuts, Wendy's, Domino's, KFC, Taco Bell, and many others.

At first, none of these highly processed and overcooked foods had much taste; it was more the idea of eating out affordably that kept people coming in. But as the market opened up, the companies experimented with ways to improve taste while keeping costs down. Salt, sugar, and fat became key components, but along with them came a variety of chemicals to mimic various flavours without containing any of the food they simulated. A book called *Fast Food Nation* tells us that a Burger King strawberry milkshake comes from a cocktail of:

amyl acetate, amyl butyrate, amyl valerate, anethol, anisyl formate, benzyl acetate, benzyl isobutyrate, butyric acide, cinnamyl isobutyrate, cinnamyl valerate, cognac essential oil, diacetyl, dipropyl ketone, ethyl acetate, ethyl amyl ketone, ethyl butyrate, ethyl cinnamate, ethyl heptanoate, ethyl heptylate, ethyl lactate, ethyl methylphenyl-glycidate, ethyl nitrate, ethy propionate, ethyl valerate, heliotropin, hydrosy[henyl-2-butanone (10 percent solution in alcohol), α-ionone, isobutyl anthranilate, isobutyl butyrate, lemon essential oil, maltol, 4-methylacetophenone, methyl anthranilate, methyl benzoate, methyl cinnamate, methyl heptine carbonate, methyl naphthyl ketone, methyl salicylate, mint essential oil, neroli essential oil, nerolin, neryl isobutyrate, orris butter, phenethyl alcohol, rose, rum ether, γ-undecalactone, vanillin, and solvent. [*]

Not a strawberry in sight.

MASS PRODUCTION AND FAST FOOD: NO COINCIDENCE

It's no coincidence that the fast food and junk food industries became a financial powerhouse at the same time as mass production of food was turning farming into agribusiness. As the largest purchaser of potatoes in the world, consuming 7.5% of America's potato crop, McDonald's has been telling many American potato farmers how to grow potatoes for a long time. This is the relationship between many fast food and junk food companies and the farmers who meet their needs.

You see, while McDonald's does not own any farms directly, its purchasing power gives it tremendous influence in the agricultural industry, not only in potato farming, but for beef, pork, and chicken farmers. Think back to Chapter 1 – if you're a farmer and you're having trouble supporting your family while competing with the big agribusiness-owned farms, one way to gain stability is by signing a contract with a company like McDonald's that will assure you of a steady income.

---

[*] *Fast Food Nation,* by Eric Schlosser, Penguin Books, 2002, http://jhampton.pbworks.com/w/file/fetch/51769044/Fast%20Food%20Nation.pdf.

In exchange, however, you'll be required to grow your potatoes to McDonald's exact specifications. McDonald's only works with farmers who grow the Russet Burbank potato because it supplies the flavour McDonald's wants. Yet the Russet Burbank is beset with so many problems that it has to be doused with chemicals just to make it to harvest.

Whether it's a company that requires farmers to raise chickens with such huge breasts they can't support their own weight, or beef pumped full of antibiotics and raised on chemical feed, the food is not grown with the consumer's health in mind. Without even considering cruelty to farm animals or the environmental impacts of chemical pesticides and fertilizers (which are horrifying but beyond the scope of this book), the extent to which fast food companies drive twenty-first century farming in the direction they choose brings me back to the 3 Ps: profit first, product second, people third.

I'll say it again: I don't believe in conspiracy theories, and I don't see any point in blaming corporations for what's going on with our health and health care system. Corporations are run by people. Among the thousands of patients I've treated over the years are people who have done all kinds of work for many different companies, and I don't believe any of those people have been involved in a conspiracy, or should be expected to take the blame for anyone's health issues but their own—and even then, I wouldn't talk about blame but rather, responsibility.

It is my job to talk about the impact of all those fast foods and junk foods on your health. It doesn't matter what you call them, their impact is all the same. It's my job to talk about the epidemic of chronic degenerative disease that's causing people to suffer needlessly and it's also my job to show how making generational health our first priority can prevent disease.

THE HIGH PRICE OF CHEAP FOOD

Fast food and junk foods may seem cheap when you buy them, but we pay a high price for them in the long term. For example, simply adding nutrients to white flour doesn't replace nutrients stripped away in the refining process. Natural nutrients occur in a matrix, which means they often work best when they work together. Refined flour also lacks fibre that's essential to effective digestion and intestinal health. Refined carbohydrates quickly turn to sugar in the blood, setting off a chain reaction that's been unequivocally linked with obesity, diabetes, heart disease, and stroke.

Processed fats are just as bad. Processing fats through hydrogenation creates nice soft margarine, but it also essentially changes fats into plastics. Where once doctors claimed margarines and cooking oils made with hydrogenated fats were heart-healthier than saturated fats, they now realize that the resulting trans-fats contribute to atherosclerosis, heart disease, and stroke. Food companies also hydrogenate cheese slices, peanut butter, mayonnaise, and shortening, and make many fried foods, packaged baked foods, and junk foods (like potato chips and cheesies) with hydrogenated fats to keep costs down.

Salt is another problem in a diet that consists of too much fast food and junk food. When all the nutrients have been refined or processed out of food, it becomes tasteless, and that taste has to be replaced. Just like the strawberry milkshake without a single strawberry, a bag of cheesies might not contain even a smidgeon of cheese.

What it does contain, in addition to a long list of chemicals that simulate the taste of cheese, is salt, and lots of it, as does every other bag of junk food on the convenience store shelf and every French fry, onion ring, chicken finger, burger, potato patty, or fish stick, and (unless it's marked low-sodium) every can of vegetables, tin of tuna, or jar of pickles. Yet health research has been telling us for years that too much salt can contribute to hypertension, which is better known as high blood pressure, which can be as deadly as heart disease and stroke.

Take a look back at the Introduction to the book, where I provided a list of statistics from the World Health Organization on the increasing rates of cardiovascular disease, various cancers, and diabetes just since 2000, and the predicted increases up to the year 2030. The low price we're paying for cheap food is actually quite high when you consider the high cost of the resulting illnesses caused by its consumption. Research is now showing strong relationships between fast food and degenerative neurological diseases including Alzheimer's, Parkinson's, and ALS, which were long thought of as diseases of aging, as well as mental illnesses, such as depression and eating disorders. I'll talk about that, not in the next chapter, but in Chapter 4.

ROLL OVER, HIPPOCRATES

Hippocrates would roll over in his grave to know the price we're paying for cheap food. He'd also likely ask, *why?* The answer, of course, is the 3 Ps. Food companies need to make profits to satisfy shareholders, so they develop products that promise great taste, fast preparation, and low prices, without considering the long-term impacts on the health of the people who buy them, because that's not their responsibility. It's ours.

It's when we don't take our responsibilities seriously that the profits begin to be shared with another industry: pharmaceutical companies. In the health care system that's evolved since World War II, we have given the pharmaceutical industry increasing responsibility for taking care of people after they get sick. And large pharmaceutical corporations operate according to the same principles as other corporations, which can be summed up by the 3 Ps. That's what I'll talk about in Chapter 3.

CHAPTER 3:
HOW DID DRUGS BECOME SUCH A BIG PART OF HEALTH?

In the Introduction to the book, I described how my classmates and I used to go on "field trips" across town, over the bridge, and up the hill to the medical school to debate with the allopathic students there. The debate I remember most clearly is the one about antibiotics.

Nearly 30 years later, allopathic doctors have become just as aware as naturopathic doctors that over-prescribing antibiotics is a bad idea. The world is now seeing the terrible consequences that we, as naturopathic students, predicted.

The truth is they're not the only ones who've softened their extreme opinions. I'm not as opposed to prescription drugs as I once was. In fact, in British Columbia, Canada, where I practice, prescribing many drugs is now within an ND's scope of practice.

This surprises many patients, such as a young man who came to me recently with a severe chest infection.

"I want you to treat it naturally," he said. "I'm aware of the issues with antibiotics and I don't want to be part of the problem."

"All right," I said. "Let's start with a detailed history."

Typically, an initial visit with a naturopathic doctor can take up to an hour, because everything starts with a detailed history. This patient's history showed, among other things, that he was generally very healthy and had good immune function.

"So what can I do about this infection?" He asked toward the end of the hour.

"I think you need antibiotics," I said.

"What!" He said, coughing. "I don't believe in antibiotics, or Big Pharma. If I'd wanted that, I would have gone to an allopathic doctor. You're a naturopathic doctor. How can you even suggest that?"

"You clearly have good eating and exercise habits," I said. "You're not on any long-term medications, and your history gives me no reason to suspect you're experiencing early symptoms of chronic disease. In naturopathy, we always try to treat underlying problems first, with a goal of preventing chronic disease, rather than going straight to palliative care. But there isn't always anything to prevent.
"

"What do you mean there's nothing to prevent?" He said, coughing. "I'm obviously sick!"

"Exactly," I said. "In your case, I have no reason to think you're at risk and require preventive care. Going by your history, your infection is an isolated incident. If you'd had multiple infections all year long and had been prescribed several courses of antibiotics, I'd want to dig deeper. But sometimes prescription drugs are the best course of action. The key is to know when to choose prevention and when to choose palliation. And you, my friend, need palliation."

THE WAR AND DRUGS

The roots of the pharmaceutical industry can't be traced back to the Industrial Revolution. Pharmaceutical companies didn't really start appearing until the late nineteenth and early twentieth century. They set out to manufacture things like vitamins, laxatives, and toothpastes. Many struggled to survive the Great Depression, but several companies made their mark during World War II.

One of the most urgent medical issues during World War II was how to treat infection. Scottish scientist Alexander Fleming discovered penicillin in 1928, but had not found a way to use it as a drug or mass produce it. After America entered the war in 1941, the government urged drug companies to take Fleming's research further as their contribution to the war effort.

Coincidentally, before the war, the pharmaceutical company Pfizer had developed a technique to manufacture vitamin C in large quantities. By 1944, Pfizer had adapted this technique to mass-producing penicillin. The massive amounts of the drug that Pfizer sent ashore with Allied Forces on D-Day, and for the rest of the war, saved countless lives. That positioned the company for rapid post-war growth, and since then it has developed and patented thousands of drugs, some of which have been important in overcoming serious diseases, such as polio in the 1960s. Pfizer is now one of the largest pharmaceutical companies in the world.

Squibb is another company that supplied penicillin to the Allies, though it's better known for a different contribution to the war effort: the Syrette. The Syrette was like a miniature toothpaste tube containing a single dose of morphine. A medic would inject the morphine under the skin of the wounded soldier and then pin the empty Syrette to the soldier's collar to show how much morphine had been administered. This alleviated suffering on the battlefield and protected soldiers against accidental overdose. After the war Squibb, like Pfizer, developed many important medicines, such as an antibiotic to fight tuberculosis.

With credentials like these, Pfizer and Squibb established strong alliances with medical schools, medical journals, and doctors themselves. Past medical practices were dismissed as old-fashioned and drugs became the method of choice to treat an ever-growing list of ailments. This was a revolutionary concept and pharmaceutical companies, with virtually unlimited funds to develop and distribute new drugs, embraced it.

WHO KNOWS?

So you wouldn't argue with the need for prescription medicines to battle life-threatening illnesses or manage pain from horrific injuries, would you?

No, of course not.

"Of course not?"

Okay, you're right. When I was in naturopathic college, we were arguing that. By the time I graduated and started my practice, I had changed my mind and by now so have most of my colleagues.

You're saying that naturopathic and allopathic care should be integrated. So does that mean they'd all become part of the same profession?

Perhaps eventually, but at this time, no, because we, as naturopathic doctors, come at health care from a different perspective than Allopaths, and it's the combination of perspectives that's most valuable to patients.

For example?

For example, I question the appropriateness of using drugs to treat a wide range of health concerns, many of which are not the result of a sudden health crisis or trauma but of years of poor food choices, not enough exercise, too much stress, and sometimes over-use of drugs.

Over-use of drugs fosters a belief that people can do whatever they wish to their bodies and then, when problems arise, the quick fix will always be there waiting for them, just take a drug or have a surgery and you will be good as new.

It's also important to understand that every drug has a range of effects in the body. Some of them are designed to combat the problem for which they're prescribed, while others have adverse effects (side effects) that can cause new health problems – sometimes worse than the conditions the drugs were meant to treat. The aspiring law student with stress-related migraines from back in my days at naturopathic college is a good example of a patient who was incorrectly diagnosed and then over-medicated to the extent that the drugs had become a large part of the problem.

Another example was a senior patient of mine who had been on a cholesterol-lowering drug for many years. Statin drugs for lowering cholesterol are among the most prescribed of drugs for chronic conditions. But because they're prescribed preventively, patients can often take them for years, often putting up with side effects such as changes in liver function, severe aching and tremors in muscles, and problems with memory, depression, and irritability. They do this without even knowing whether the drug is benefiting them. A recent newspaper article noted that some doctors are now saying that, when you take into account all the groups of people with risk factors, one in every three adults need these drugs to control their cholesterol levels. That is a beggar's belief considering there is little evidence that statins prevent heart attacks and strokes in most people. It's no wonder the new recommendations have triggered a backlash and led to questions about whether cardiologists have put prescribing drugs ahead of preventing heart disease.[*]

---

[*] "It's Time to Question the New Guidelines on Cholesterol Drugs," by André Picard, *The Globe and Mail,* November 24, 2013, http://www.theglobeandmail.com/life/health-and-

The problem is two-fold. First, patients are simply told that the drug reduces cholesterol levels by 50% and therefore helps protect them against heart disease. Heart disease is one of the most lethal of the killer diseases plaguing us today, so they do what their doctor says. Second, allopathic doctors don't always know as much as we think they do about the drugs they're prescribing.

In fact, a 2013 study at the University of British Columbia suggested doctors often know little about many of the drugs they prescribe. As one doctor said, "doctors learn relatively little about drugs in medical school, and much of their exposure to pharmacology after graduation may be in the form of advertising. If they are unaware of the potential harms from drugs they prescribe, patients inevitably suffer the consequences."[†]

So doctors learn about drugs from advertising—the same advertising we see on TV?

Not exactly. The study says doctors often get most of their information about a drug from pharmaceutical company sales representatives. Sales representatives are legally required to disclose full information about the drugs they're selling to doctors, but they don't always get the chance. Doctors tend to be very busy people. When they have a waiting room full of patients who are ill or who have schedules of their own or who are minding cranky children, they may be squeezing those meetings with sales representatives into a few short minutes in a backlog of patients.

ABSOLUTE AND RELATIVE RISK

There's sometimes also an issue with the way drug companies describe research results. Researchers think of risk in two ways: absolute and relative. Say a company does a study of a cholesterol-lowering drug. Often studies include thousands of people, but for simplicity I'll say there are 100 people involved in this study who may be at risk of heart attack due to a combination of cholesterol levels, personal or family history, and other factors, but only six of

---

fitness/health/its-time-to-question-the-new-guidelines-on-cholesterol-drugs/article15566990/.

† "Doctors Not Informed of Harmful Effects of Medicines during Sales Visits," UBC Public Affairs media release, April 10, 2013, http://www.publicaffairs.ubc.ca/2013/04/10/doctors-not-informed-of-harmful-effects-of-medicines-during-sales-visits/.

those 100 people have actually had a coronary episode. Of those six, only three have a coronary episode during the study, while taking the drug.

There are now two ways to interpret the risk. If we speak about absolute risk, we look at total numbers. Out of 100 people with risk factors, 6% were really at risk, and 3% benefitted from the drug. So prevention of absolute risk is only 3%. But if we look at relative risk, of the six people who were really at risk, three benefited from the drug, and therefore that's a 50% reduction in relative risk.

When it comes to selling the drug, the company will say the study showed a 50% reduction in risk of heart attack among study participants who had a combination of high cholesterol and other risk factors, and therefore all people with high cholesterol and other risk factors (which could just mean a grandfather had heart disease) should take this drug.

Isn't that called "manipulating the data"?

No. It's just using it selectively. So when the sales representative goes into the doctor's office and tries to fit her pitch into the few minutes the doctor can spare, she may very well rhyme off the same long list of possible side effects that we hear when we watch the TV advertisement about the same drug. But if the focus of the pitch is on a 50% reduction in relative risk of heart attack, what the doctor is most likely to hear is that the benefits of this drug far outweigh the risk of side effects.

Shouldn't we expect our doctors to get more education in medical school, or stay sufficiently abreast of research to question these numbers?

I don't think that's realistic. Every doctor has hundreds of patients to keep track of, and thousands of drugs, with the numbers increasing every day. They're not superheroes. They're human. There are limits to what we should expect of them. And blaming them is no better than blaming corporations. The responsibility for your health lies with you.

WORKING WITH SYSTEMS

There's even more to it than that, allopathic doctors work within a system. In allopathic medicine that system is called "differential diagnosis." When a patient describes symptoms, the doctor makes a list (usually mentally), compares it with a list of possible causes, orders tests to rule out the most dangerous causes, and treats the most likely causes. The doctor chooses treatments according to accepted protocols based on scientific evidence that has been gathered and tested according to rigorous standards.

If the protocol is that a patient with high cholesterol levels should be prescribed cholesterol-lowering drugs, the doctor is more than likely to follow the protocol. In the worst case scenario, if a doctor fails to follow established protocols and patients worsen or die, he may have little protection against a malpractice suit, or he may even lose his license to practice, and he can't do much good for his patients then.

So even if the doctor has some questions about a certain protocol, the system discourages acting upon it until and unless the protocols change. That's one reason why it's so important for you to become informed and accountable for your own health—so you can decide when to go to which professional for what kind of care.

I thought you weren't judging systems.

I'm not criticizing the system of allopathic medicine any more than I'm criticizing corporate influence. The system of differential diagnosis and treatment has evolved over many years and, like everything else, there are good points and bad points about it. The goal of using differential diagnosis and prescribing evidence-based treatment protocols is to protect patients by ensuring all doctors are working to the same standards of care based on the same quality of research. That's a good thing.

Naturopaths are also taught to use 'differential diagnosis', but as a result of our naturopathic training our approach provides more creative treatment options to our patients. It's more geared toward prevention than palliation, but it also has it's limitations. Back when I was a student and a young doctor, I had only begun to question the limitations of the naturopathic system. But after nearly 30 years of practice, it's clear to me that both systems have situations in which they work well and others in which they don't. I believe the doctor of the future will recognize that appropriate intervention in health can be either naturopathic or allopathic. The doctor of the future will integrate both disciplines – and perhaps others, as well.

RESPONSIBILITY, NOT BLAME

But let's get back to my senior patient. She'd been on cholesterol-lowering medications for years. She was suffering a range of side effects. But when I did some testing I found that, although her total cholesterol level was high, her ratio of good to bad cholesterol, which is the most important measure of cholesterol levels, was within a good range.

She had no other risk factors for heart attack, yet she'd been prescribed a cholesterol-lowering drug and told she'd need to take it for the rest of her life. This is another reason why it's so important for patients to become informed and accountable for their own health – so they'll know where to find information for themselves, what kinds of questions to ask their doctors, and sometimes when to seek a second opinion in order to ensure that they're getting the health care that's right for them. For example, progressive minded doctors are using the "Framingham" coronary heart disease risk assessment, before recommending any drug therapy to reduce mortality or morbidity rates.

When this patient first came to the clinic and I explained all this to her, she was shocked to learn that this drug had been shown to have little to no impact on mortality rates unless the patient had a history of heart disease, and that even then the impact on mortality was at best 4%. She was angry to think of all the years she'd been suffering side effects that she need not have suffered.

Wasn't she right to be angry?

Maybe, but I don't think that would have helped her or anyone else. No one in our health care system acts alone, and that's a good thing. Just as plenty of good has come over the years from the economic system that grew out of the Industrial Revolution, plenty of good comes out of our health care system everyday, but no system is perfect. People within any system are just doing their jobs. If anyone is responsible, it's the individual who needs to be accountable for becoming informed so they can make truly informed choices.

GET INFORMED CONSENT

Fortunately, it's become very easy to do that. During the late 1980s and early 1990s, when I was beginning my practice, we were all introduced to the World Wide Web. Since then, medicine has never been the same. Patients now have the ability to be almost as informed as their doctors, at least on the matters that pertain to their particular health issues.

Yes, there's a lot of bad information on the Internet, but there's also good information. For example, pharmaceutical companies post profiles of all their drugs online, and those profiles are accurate. They show the good and the bad. Getting full information on a drug before you take it is an important aspect of informed consent.

Ideally, except in cases of acute illness or injury, patients should seek out information about their health before going to either an allopath or a naturopath, because they should understand that their health begins with them. They should recognize that over several generations we've lost control of our health in many different ways, and now we need to take it back. That's what I'll start talking about in the next chapter with a look at how we lost control of body composition.

CHAPTER 4:
HOW DID WE LOSE CONTROL OF OUR BODY COMPOSITION?

Like all parents, I'm proud of my children. One thing I'm especially proud of is their attitude towards food, and especially fast food or junk food.

You might think, as a naturopath, I wouldn't allow my kids to eat anything but "natural" foods, but I've always believed that there's a time and a place for everything; we just need to understand how things work so we can use them to our benefit. As a parent myself, I understand how busy life can be, rushing kids from school to their soccer game, rushing back home for dinner, and then rushing out to a parent-teacher meeting, for example.

Occasionally, when life is busy, it's not a bad idea to choose fast foods or convenience foods. Which would you rather do – grab something quick at the drive-through and have a little time to spend with your kids in a busy day, or spend every minute of your free time cooking and cleaning up while your children are doing their homework or watching TV?

I don't have a problem if my patients, or my own children, eat some of the foods they know aren't the best nutritionally once in a while, as long as they're not doing it all the time, there's no reason for it to be a problem.

My son said something to me recently that made me proud to see he's gotten that message.

"Dad," he said. "Do you know I sometimes go with my friends to the local fast food restaurant and get a burger and fries?"

"Yes, I know that," I said. "There's nothing wrong with that, as long as it's an occasional treat."

"Yeah, it is," he said. "You don't have to worry about that."

"That's good," I said. "But something seems to be bothering you."

"I'm kind of worried about some of my friends," he said. "Some of them go to McDonald's for lunch or after school every day – sometimes even twice in one day. I don't know how they can do that."

"Yeah, you'd think they'd get tired of it," I said.

"Not just tired of it," he said. "I'd think they'd feel sick. I mean, I like a burger once in a while, but I think eating a burger and fries every day would just make me feel disgusting."

"Me too," I said.

He stopped and thought about it for a minute, and then he said something that suggested he's developing a lot of insight at a young age.

"I wonder if they eat it so often they don't know what it's like to feel any other way," he said.

"That's quite possible," I said. "I see it in my practice all the time. It's sad, but it's possible."

REFINED SUGAR: A LEGAL ADDICTION

You might think my son and I were over-dramatizing the situation, talking about his friends eating McDonald's as if fast food were some kind of serious addiction to hard drugs. But that's exactly the point – they are. People who eat unhealthy diets all the time don't recognize that they don't feel well because they can't remember or never knew what it was like to feel any other way. They're addicted to fast food or junk food in exactly the same way they could be addicted to drugs or alcohol.

Although highly processed foods are filled with chemical flavours, colours, and preservatives whose impacts on health remain uncertain, the biggest health problems derive from three primary ingredients: sugar, fat, and salt. Compelling research shows that refined sugar, hydrogenated fat, and refined salt all have powerful addictive properties that make it tremendously difficult to "kick the habit."

The first researchers to prove refined sugar is addictive did their groundbreaking studies at Princeton University in 2008. A study in rats showed refined sugar changed brain chemistry in much the same way that cocaine, morphine, and nicotine do. The changes were so powerful that even the rats' inclination to consume other drugs, such as alcohol, was increased.

This is because sugar increases levels of a brain chemical called dopamine, which controls the brain's pleasure centre. Previous studies had demonstrated similar changes in rats that had been addicted to cocaine and heroin. Moreover, when the rats' sugar was taken away, they displayed typical symptoms of withdrawal.

Research in humans has used brain scans to confirm sugar is just as addictive as alcohol, cocaine, morphine, and heroin. In a 2012 segment on the TV show 60 Minutes, Dr. Sanjay Gupta lay inside an fMRI scanner at the Oregon Research Institute while a straw delivered a tiny drop of sweet soda to his mouth. "Just as it hit my tongue," he said, "the scanner detected increased blood rushing to certain regions of my brain [which caused dopamine to be released], just as it would in response to drugs or alcohol."[*]

In the quantities of sugar many people consume, which some research suggests may be as much as one-third of a pound daily, such rapid dopamine release triggers an immediate sense of euphoria. By scanning hundreds of volunteers, the Oregon researchers observed that people who eat or drink a lot of sugar seem to develop a tolerance: the more they eat, the less they feel the reward, and the more they need to eat. This is the same process that leads to drug addiction.

A third of a pound of sugar a day? You must be talking about people with eating disorders.

No, I'm not. It's easy for people who don't have eating disorders, such as obesity or bulimia, to judge those who do as having no willpower, but this research tells us that it's just as difficult to kick a sugar addiction as a drug, alcohol, or nicotine. And a lot of people who don't have eating disorders struggle with the same addictions.

In fact, in some ways, a sugar addiction can be worse than a drug addiction. A drug addict can avoid things that trigger cravings, but a sugar addict is besieged by advertising that assaults everyone's

---

[*] "Sugar," by Dr. Sanjay Gupta, *60 Minutes,* aired on CNN Apr 1, 2012. Posted October 29, 2012 as "Sugar Exposé, 60 Minutes, Dr. Sanjay Gupta" on *YouTube* at https://www.youtube.com/watch?v=HezSlrJ1k7w.

will power every day with images of tantalizing treats that are completely legal and available in any corner store and most kitchen cupboards.

Children in many families grow up with a sugar addiction from the time they are very small, drinking fruit juice out of bottles, gobbling candy at Halloween, Christmas, and Easter, and running to the ice cream truck in the summer. That addiction builds throughout childhood and continues into adulthood, when parents pass it along to their own children. This then contributes to the current epidemics of obesity and related health issues like diabetes, hypertension, heart disease, and cancer.

Is this what you're talking about when you use the term "Generational Health First"?

Exactly, but we're getting ahead of ourselves. Even if the sugar addict learns to avoid the obvious sugars, hidden sugars lurk in almost every processed or convenience food. Addicts might not even realize how much sugar they're still eating or why they're continually relapsing because it often appears in ingredient lists under another name, such as high-fructose corn syrup. When food corporations first came out with high-fructose corn syrup, they said it was natural and healthier than sugar, but high-fructose corn syrup behaves the same way in your body as any refined sugar.

The key word here is "refined." Your body needs sugar to create energy. It powers your muscles and converts any excess sugar into fat for you to burn when blood sugar levels run down. But the human body didn't evolve to deal with sugar that's been so heavily refined that it's absorbed the second it hits the tongue. Throughout evolution, we got our sugar from fruits and vegetables, which include fibre that slows down digestion and ensures sugar is released into the body in small amounts. As it became less expensive to refine sugar, we started eating more and more of it. Now it's become one of many factors in our current obesity epidemic.[†]

[†] "Why We Should Consider Obesity a Disease," by Dr. Arya Sharma, *The Globe and Mail,* Jan 19, 2014, http://www.theglobeandmail.com/life/health-and-fitness/health-advisor/why-we-should-consider-obesity-a-disease/article16370893/

DISEASES RELATED TO REFINED SUGAR

From obesity, it's not a big leap to other degenerative health problems ranging from diabetes and heart disease to cancer. Diabetes occurs when the body either lacks enough insulin or develops insulin resistance. Insulin regulates delivery of blood sugar into cells to provide them with energy, and also ensures blood sugar levels do not go too high, which can cause diabetic coma and even death.

In Type I diabetes, which is usually at least partly genetic, the pancreas cannot produce enough insulin to meet the body's needs. In Type II diabetes, the pancreas produces insulin but the body's cells have developed insulin resistance because the patient has lived on a diet high in sugar (including refined starches, like white flour) for too long.

It's only in the last few decades, as Type II diabetes has increasingly surfaced in younger adults, teenagers, and now children, that the names for these conditions have changed from juvenile diabetes and adult-onset diabetes to Types I and II diabetes. This shows how quickly diabetes has reached epidemic proportions, and there is no doubt it is connected with the rapid rise in obesity.

It's long been known that diabetes is a leading contributor to heart disease, and current studies illustrate the nature of that connection. In one ongoing study, volunteers are kept on a sugar-restricted diet for several days, and then switched to a diet with the same number of calories but including sugary drinks. Researchers take blood samples every 30 minutes, which have shown that blood levels of LDL cholesterol (the bad cholesterol) increase dramatically within two weeks of this change.

High cholesterol is a result of increasing sugar in the diet? I thought fat was the big factor in heart disease.

Back in the 1970s, that's what health researchers told us, and governments responded by launching a very successful public health campaign. From a corporate perspective, this was a great thing as it created a demand for whole new lines of low-fat and fat-free products. However, decreasing fat content also decreased flavour, so companies replaced fat with sugar, but instead of reducing the frequency of heart disease, the opposite happened – rates of heart disease soared.

Communicating this new information to the public has been difficult. One expert interviewed on *60 Minutes* said that even many medical doctors are unaware of this research. Even less well known is that sugar has become a focus in cancer research, too, because cells in some types of cancer have learned to hijack blood glucose away from its mission to provide energy, instead shipping it directly to cancer cells where it helps tumours grow.

That's scary!

Yes, it is. It's every bit as scary as the truth about fats.

FATS: THE GOOD, THE BAD, AND THE DEADLY

Fats are not our enemy. Just as your body needs sugar, it needs fat; what it doesn't need is processed fat. Like refined sugar, processed fat can be addictive, especially when it's combined with refined sugar. However, research suggests refined fats have their own addictive qualities. Let's start with understanding why we need fat, and how the damage caused by the low-fat campaign goes beyond the damage of substituting sugars for fats in low-fat products.

The fats we need to survive are called essential fatty acids (EFA), also known as omega-3 and omega-6. These fats (*cis*-fats) spoil quickly, so as agriculture, food corporations, and fast-food restaurants moved toward mass-producing food and shipping it long distances to supermarkets and fast-food franchises, food companies developed a process called hydrogenation to prevent spoilage and extend shelf life. This process involves adding hydrogen to liquid vegetable fats to make them solidify. However, it also alters the molecular structure of fat so dramatically that it more closely resembles plastic than natural fat.

When hydrogenation came into widespread use in the 1950s and 1960s, people weren't thinking about whether they should eat a product that, under a microscope, looked like plastic, all they knew or cared about was that margarine stayed soft in the fridge, cooking oil didn't need to be refrigerated, and shortening gave cakes, cookies, and pastries a melt-in-your-mouth texture.

As well, hydrogenated fats (trans-fats) can be made from inexpensive sources, like corn, coconuts, and palm trees. This sounded healthy, so it became another selling point. Hydrogenated fats were also unsaturated, and at the time saturation was considered the crucial factor that made fats bad. Not least of all, because hydrogenated fats didn't spoil, budget-conscious families could buy them in bulk and they'd last almost indefinitely. Hydrogenated fats generated almost limitless profits, gave rise to numerous products, and people believed they were good for their health.

HYDROGENATED FATS: THE DISEASES THEY CAN CAUSE

As it turned out, although everything else was true, hydrogenated fats are not good for your health. In fact, they're killers. Trans-fats do two important things that contribute almost immeasurably to increasing risk of heart disease:

- Trans-fats raise blood levels of so-called bad cholesterols (LDL cholesterol). A high blood level of LDL cholesterol is a risk factor for heart disease.
- Trans-fats lower blood levels of so-called good cholesterol (HDL cholesterol). A high blood level of HDL cholesterol protects against heart disease.

Both LDL and HDL cholesterol serve important roles in your body; research has shown it's almost pointless to measure cholesterol levels without measuring levels of LDL and HDL relative to each other. The important thing is balance.

So as long as we eat trans-fats in balance, it's all good?

Yes and no. Trans-fats are one area of health where balance means next to nothing; they're almost always bad for you. Trans-fats occur only rarely in nature, and natural trans-fats don't appear to cause the same damage as artificial trans-fats because our bodies have evolved ways to metabolize them. This is not true of processed fats.

Research suggests a diet high in hydrogenated fats may cause obesity even when a person is not eating a high-calorie diet overall. Obesity is always a risk factor for heart disease and diabetes. And being either obese or diabetic increases the risk of developing heart disease.

But heart disease is not the only serious health issue directly linked with consuming hydrogenated fats. High levels of trans-fats can also increase the risk of infertility in both women and men. And trans-fats combined with high-fructose corn syrup may be a factor in liver dysfunction.

Trans-fats may even be a factor in mental health. A 2012 study involving nearly 9,000 participants showed that people who eat commercial baked goods and fast food were 51% more likely to develop depression than those who ate little or none – and the more people consumed, the greater their risk of depression. There's barely an aspect of health that hasn't been badly affected by the introduction of trans-fats to our daily diets.

Wait a minute. Three paragraphs ago, you said, "yes **and** no." Where's the "yes" part?

Right, I lost track. As I said earlier in the chapter, if eating a burger and fries or a chocolate bar once in a while helps you sustain good habits the rest of the time, or allows you to reduce your stress level by squeezing in a little time with your kids on a busy day, an occasional self-indulgence is not going to hurt. You just can't ever think it's safe to eat them more than once in a while.

Okay. But what about saturated fats? Weren't they the reason for the public health campaign back in the 1970s?

Yes. In the 1970s, researchers believed saturated fats were the culprits in rising rates of heart disease, and that was the main impetus behind the public health campaign, which was what drove us down the trans-fat road to begin with. It's ironic that, in addition to the mountains of information that researchers have piled up against hydrogenation, recent studies suggest saturated fat is not the villain we thought it was.

The highly respected *British Medical Journal* recently published an editorial saying "it is time to bust the myth of the role of saturated [fat] in heart disease and wind back the harms of dietary advice that has contributed to obesity," because one study after another has failed to show that a low-fat diet reduces the risk of heart attack or stroke. Moreover, the author adds, "Doctors need to embrace prevention as well as treatment."[‡]

SALT: WHY SO MUCH IN OUR DIET?

Sugar and fats are not the only areas where we got it wrong. Salt is another big one. Like sugar and fat, salt (in moderation) is essential to health. Salt contains sodium and chloride, which are electrolytes. Electrolytes, as their name implies, conduct electrical impulses to the nerves, contract and relax muscles, and maintain the proper balance of water and minerals in our bodies.

However, most Americans consume about 1.5 to 2 teaspoons of salt per day, about 3,500 milligrams. That's far more than the daily recommended limit of 2,300 milligrams per day. As with sugar, though, even when we think we're not eating a lot of salt, we often are, because food corporations add so much to processed foods. Here are a few foods that are surprisingly high in sodium:

- Kellogg's Raisin Bran: 350 mg of sodium in one cup of cereal (15% of daily limit).
- Kellogg's Eggo Buttermilk Pancakes: 580 mg of sodium in three pancakes (25% of daily limit).
- Kraft Singles: 200 mg of sodium in a single slice (almost one-third of daily limit).
- Heinz Ketchup: 190 mg of sodium in a single tablespoon (16% of daily recommended limit).
- Duncan Hines Moist Deluxe Devil's Food Cake Mix: 380 mg of sodium in a slice that equals one-twelfth of the whole cake (15% of daily limit).
- Friendship 1% Low-Fat Cottage Cheese: 360 mg of sodium in a half-cup serving (15% of daily limit).
- Bertolli Mediterranean Style Shrimp and Penne Primavera: 890 mg of sodium in half of a 24-ounce package (more than one-third of daily recommended limit).

---

‡ "Observations: Saturated Fat is not the Major Issue," *British Medical Journal*, Oct 22, 2013, http://www.bmj.com/press-releases/2013/10/22/observations-saturated-fat-not-major-issue.

- Bird's Eye Asian Vegetable in Sesame Ginger Sauce contains 630 mg of sodium in just one cup (25% of daily recommended limit).
- Otis Spunkmeyer Harvest Bran Muffin: 420 mg of sodium in a single muffin (over 20% of daily limit).

Really? In a bran muffin? And a vegetable stir-fry? Why is so much salt added to our food?

Salt sells. People love salt. And salt, too, is habit forming. An article in *Slate* describes high salt consumption as having a "quasi-addictive effect." I wouldn't call it "quasi-addictive." The more salt you eat, the more you want. The article goes on to say that,

> *In 2011 researchers at Philadelphia's Monell Chemical Senses Center, the source of many salt consumption studies, found that babies who eat salty, starchy foods almost immediately begin to crave salt at higher levels than their salt-naïve peers. There are even indications from rodent studies that a mother's salt intake, transmitted to her baby in her breast milk, can affect its salt cravings later in life. Perhaps even more importantly for the processed food industry, people who lower their sodium intake for just two to three months experience a measurable decrease in salt cravings.[δ]*

So there's a good reason for food manufacturers to want you to keep on eating salt. Too many customers kicking the salt habit would not be good for profits. Salt makes food taste good, so we want to eat more of all those foods that are so bad for us, and salt makes us thirsty, which is what makes soft drinks seem like such a perfect partner for salty chips.

SALT: ARE REFINED AND UNREFINED REALLY THE SAME?

All of this research, however, has focused on refined salt. Unrefined salt barely enters the discussion. Knowing how badly refinement impacts sugars and fats, why would we expect refining salt to be any less damaging? In fact, unrefined salt can contain over 80 trace

---

[δ] "Why Is There So Much Salt in Processed Foods?" by Brian Palmer, May 15, 2013, *Slate,* http://www.slate.com/articles/health_and_science/explainer/2013/05/salt_dietary_guideline s_why_do_food_manufacturers_use_so_much_salt.html.

minerals, depending on where it is mined, and all of them are important to health. The refining process removes these trace minerals, leaving only sodium and chloride behind.

Dr. David Brownstein, an MD who converted to a holistic practice, noticed that after he began recommending unrefined salt to his patients, even those who had suffered from hypertension for a long time had lower blood pressure. The conventional wisdom is that too much salt can cause hypertension, heart disease, and stroke, but when Brownstein looked into it, he found research that reviewed 57 studies and revealed "almost no change in patients with normal blood pressure who ate a low-salt diet."[♦]

But that's not the same as proving it's okay for people with high blood pressure to eat high-salt diets.

No. It's not good for anyone to eat too much salt, refined or not. It's not good to eat too much of any one thing, but it reminds me that back in the 1970s the conventional wisdom was that saturated fats were at the root of heart disease. Apparently, accepting the conventional wisdom doesn't always work out very well. We have to keep asking questions, because sometimes research isn't as conclusive as we thought it was.

So why is salt refined? Don't say it... the 3 Ps?

Right. First, profit: salt, like sugar and fat, can spoil if perishable properties are not removed. Refinement allows for it to remain on a shelf without an expiry date, which helps salt producers avoid financial losses.

Second, product: salt in its natural state takes on different colours, like gray, pink, and even red, depending on the combinations of trace minerals it includes. But manufacturers think bright white salt looks cleaner and will therefore be a more appealing product to customers.

Third, people: the salt-refining industry sells its product to people by claiming it's healthier than unrefined salt. For example, if the salt comes from a heavily polluted area, refining can remove pollutants. This is true, but perhaps it should just not be mined from

---

[♦] "Are You Salt Deficient?" by Dr. David Brownstein, *Caduseus*, issue 79, pages 16–19.

those areas. (Maybe that would even be a good reason to clean those areas up, though that's not my area of expertise.)

More importantly, the salt-refining industry says the iodine they add to table salt is essential to our health. It's true our bodies need iodine, and refined salt contains more iodine than unrefined salt, but the amount of iodine added to salt isn't enough to meet our bodies' needs. We also don't know if the kind that's added (because there's more than one) is the most bioavailable kind (which means most easily absorbed by our bodies). So the argument in favour of iodized salt doesn't seem very substantial.

THE OBSTACLES TO PHYSICAL FITNESS

Let's go back, briefly, to the Industrial Revolution. Before it began, people did all labour manually. Every aspect of life, from tilling the fields and keeping the house to traveling from one place to another required physical effort. The inventions of the Industrial Revolution began to change that, but even those early innovations demanded far more exertion than most people in the industrial world could tolerate on a daily basis today.

It's only been in the 70 years since World War II that the amount of physical exertion required to get through a day has diminished so dramatically that it may now be as significant a factor in developing most chronic degenerative diseases as processed foods and overeating. It was only the late 1940s that researchers made the first direction link between lack of exercise and development of chronic disease. It began with a British study showing that, all other factors equal, bus drivers, who sat all day, were at greater risk of heart attack than bus conductors, who were on their feet all day.

The fact that this connection was discovered so recently seems surprising until you realize that, of course, that was when all the factors that have led to our problems with body composition and chronic disease began to converge. After the war, mass food production led to an over-abundant food supply, the likes of which humanity had never seen. The advent of commercial television in the 1950s encouraged everyone to want all the new labour-saving devices, from cars to dishwashers, as well as the new convenience foods that no one yet knew were deadly.

By the 1960s, once fast food was becoming more established and labour-saving devices were reducing physical exertion, there was a slight bump in the overall weight of the population, and people like TV fitness pioneer Jack LaLanne took the opportunity to encourage housewives to spend time during their day getting some exercise, but statistics suggest the obesity epidemic in adults didn't really start to until the 1970s.

Ironically, that was also when fitness movements began attracting interest. Or maybe it's not ironic. Somewhere along the line, the 3 Ps became a significant factor in fitness. Suddenly people needed fashionable outfits to attend trendy fitness classes, expensive swimsuits to go for a dip in the pool, and very pricey lift tickets, gear, and clothing to spend a day on the slopes.

The 1980s saw the introduction of home computers, and the beginning of twin addictions to electronics and junk foods. Some experts pin the start of the childhood obesity epidemic to the 1990s, when computer games and instant messaging were all the rage for children and teens – we'll talk more about children and obesity in Chapter 25.

Physical exertion is more essential to our health now than ever, but we are also far less likely than ever before to get the exercise we need. We're working so hard to earn enough money to buy all the things considered necessities of life in the twenty-first century that it's nearly impossible to find the time to keep up with most popular fitness activities, and that's not even considering the cost. It's understandable why many people get frustrated and give up on fitness when time and cost have become such enormous obstacles. Yet 70 years ago, before all our labour-saving devices and convenience foods had been invented, fitness wasn't even really an issue for most people.

I'm not an expert on the subject of exercise and fitness, and I won't go into it here in the same depth as I've explored food issues and their relationship to body composition, but in Chapter 20 I will provide some ideas for getting started with physical activity. It doesn't have to be expensive. You don't need any fancy gear or clothing. It doesn't even have to require a huge time commitment. The main thing to remember about body composition and exercise is that some type and amount of physical activity is always better than none.

BODY COMPOSITION AND THE 3 PS

Are you beginning to understand how all this connects with losing control of body composition? Today, much of our diet is made up of refined foods. The switch from whole, unprocessed foods happened gradually, before we understood their ill effects on health, and because refined foods have addictive qualities, it's difficult to give them up, even when we know they're bad for us and can see in the mirror that our bodies don't look the way we want them to.

This is why I consider education so important. Only by understanding how we got where we are, and why it's so difficult to change, do we have any hope of changing. I believe it's important to change, not only for ourselves, but for our children. Parents inevitably want something better for their children than they had for themselves. I can't think of anything better to give our children than good health. One of the best ways to do that is to kick our addictions to processed foods, not only because of what they mean for body composition, but because of the role they play in the epidemic of food intolerances we've been seeing. That's what I'll talk about in the next chapter.

CHAPTER 5:
HOW DID WE DEVELOP FOOD INTOLERANCES?

Several years ago, a 60-year-old woman came to the clinic. She had mid-stage rheumatoid arthritis (RA), walked with a cane, had visible swelling in her finger joints, and didn't sleep well because of her pain, yet she was very positive, upbeat, and motivated. She'd read that food intolerances could contribute to inflammation, and wondered if some changes to her diet might reduce her pain.

"When was this diagnosed?" I asked.

"About three years ago," she said.

"Was that when you started having symptoms?" I asked.

"Oh no," she said. "My muscles have felt tired and achy for years."

The ensuing conversation revealed there was more going on with this patient than met the eye. When she was growing up she'd often had to act like a second mother to several younger siblings. Now in her sixties, she was still caregiving her mother, though the relationship was dysfunctional and she felt perpetually stressed about money.

A physical exam showed that, in addition to the swelling in her finger joints, her knees and her elbows were inflamed, and she had reduced range of motion in all her joints. She was managing her pain with prescribed anti-inflammatory drugs, and her doctor had been regularly increasing the dosages.

"Do the drugs help?" I asked.

"Yes," she said. "But my stomach is always upset. My rheumatologist has suggested immuno-suppressive drugs to reduce the inflammation, but he also said it would cause more side effects. I read that food intolerances can cause inflammation and that naturopathy can help with food intolerances, so I came to see you."

Food intolerance testing showed aggressive reactions to gluten and eggs, and a mild reaction to dairy products. She eliminated these foods and within a few months began noticing improvements. Her joint swelling had lessened by about 15%,she was more mobile, and it hurt less to use her hands.

I'd made a good start with this patient, but there was more work to do. However, she'd come to me with the same misperception many people have about naturopathic doctors – that the only thing we do is test for food intolerances. People don't realize that, although food intolerances can cause other health issues, they can also be symptoms of other health issues. That's what I believed was going on here, but I'll get back to that in Chapter 7.

FOOD ALLERGIES AND INTOLERANCES: AN ALLOPATHIC VIEW

Allopathic and naturopathic doctors see food allergies and intolerances differently. From an allopathic perspective, food allergies happen when the immune system releases immunoglobulin E (IgE) in response to a particular food protein that it interprets as harmful. The reaction is immediate (from minutes to an hour) and triggers the release of histamine, which can cause typical allergic reactions like hives, runny nose, sneezing, wheezing, and in severe cases, anaphylaxis (blocking off of air supply).

From an allopathic perspective, a food intolerance is different than a food allergy. The allopathic perspective is that intolerances do not involve the immune system, but the digestive system. An intolerance reaction occurs when the body lacks an enzyme to digest a particular food, which then has a delayed onset (from one to four hours), and causes nausea, vomiting, abdominal cramping, or diarrhea.

Milk reactions are a good way to demonstrate the different ways allopathic medicine views allergies and intolerances: in an allergy, milk proteins trigger a release of IgE, whereas in milk intolerance, the body lacks an enzyme (lactase) to digest milk sugar (lactose). Celiac disease seems like it should be another clear example of food intolerance: it is an autoimmune disorder that occurs when the body lacks the enzyme needed to digest gluten, which is a protein.

Wait. Aren't proteins the things that cause food allergies?

Yes, but in the allopathic view, celiac disease is an intolerance, or enzymatic, reaction rather than an allergic reaction.

But isn't an allergy a reaction by the immune system rather than the digestive system?

Yes.

Doesn't "autoimmune disorder" mean it involves the immune system?

Yes.

But doesn't celiac disease, as an intolerance, involve the digestive system rather than the immune system?

That's where it becomes complicated, because the intestines are involved in immune function. In fact, the intestines are the biggest and arguably the most important organ in the immune system, because they're where food is broken down, absorbed, and transformed into all the different elements, like immunoglobulins, that make the immune system the complex and amazing thing it is. So from a naturopathic point of view, celiac disease is immunological.

But aren't food intolerances supposed to be different from allergies because they don't trigger the release of immunoglobulin E?

Yes and no. It turns out there are different kinds of food allergies, and they're classified by whether they are IgE-mediated allergies or non-IgE-mediated allergies. Some food allergies involve other immunoglobulins, specifically IgA and IgG.

What's the difference?

IgE-mediated food allergies can (but don't always) cause anaphylaxis, whereas non-IgE-mediated allergies only cause non-life-threatening reactions, like hives, itching, runny nose, and sneezing, but not anaphylaxis.

So what's an example of a non-IgE-mediated allergy?

Celiac disease.

Hold on! Didn't we just learn that, according to the allopathic view, celiac disease is not a result of food allergy, but food intolerance?

Yes, but although celiac disease is sometimes considered a food intolerance (because the body lacks enzymes such as amylase to digest gluten), other times, it's considered a food allergy (because it's due to a non-IgE-mediated immune response).

That's confusing.

Yes, it is.

Does that mean it's wrong?

No. Health research is ongoing. We're always learning and improving our understanding. Sometimes that means confirming what we thought was true, or finding it wasn't entirely true, or realizing it was completely untrue, like our understanding of the role of fats in heart disease or the dangers of overusing antibiotics. Allopathic and naturopathic medicine look at food allergies and intolerances differently, but either way, our understanding of unusual reactions to food is in its infancy. If nothing else, a naturopathic perspective is a little less confusing.

FOOD ALLERGIES AND INTOLERANCES:

A NATUROPATHIC VIEW

In naturopathic medicine, we see all food reactions as intolerances. Whether an intolerant response is coming from immune system or the digestive system, it's still a sign that the body is reacting to the food by trying to get rid of it. It's a single problem that occurs on a spectrum. People can progress from sensitivity (which allopathic medicine defines as milder than intolerance) to intolerance, and then to allergy.

Remember the term "differential diagnosis" from Chapter 3? Allopathic doctors need a diagnosis, or at least a strong suspicion of one, to prescribe a treatment. Think about a mother taking her little boy to the doctor with eczema so bad he's scratched his skin raw. He can't sleep at night, and his mom is at her wit's end. An allopathic doctor would likely diagnose eczema, for which the accepted protocol is cortisone cream. That might be the end of it, unless the condition didn't resolve, at which point the allopathic doctor would likely refer the little boy to a dermatologist, or maybe an allergist.

In the early days of my practice, I might have suggested putting the boy in an oatmeal bath daily and giving him evening primrose oil, because both contain GLA, a fatty acid effective in treating eczema, but they both take time to work. In the meanwhile, the child is suffering. At this point, I'd prescribe cortisone cream to relieve the immediate symptoms, but I'd also want to explore underlying causes, so I'd proceed to food testing. If that didn't clear the eczema up, I'd look for causes underlying the food intolerances.

Do allopathic and naturopathic doctors see everything about food intolerance differently?

No. We all agree that food intolerance is on the rise, affecting anywhere from 2% to 20% of the population. The huge range in those numbers illustrates one of the differences between the allopathic and naturopathic views. The smaller number has generally been confirmed through allopathic diagnostic techniques, while the larger number is from patients who report their own symptoms as intolerances without allopathic confirmation.

An allopathic doctor needs to confirm what a patient is reporting before prescribing a treatment. If she can't confirm a diagnosis, she probably won't prescribe a treatment, and the patient may walk away frustrated. A naturopathic doctor assumes that if patients are self-reporting symptoms allopathic tests can't confirm, the patient is at the mild end of the food intolerance spectrum. Our goal is to prevent those symptoms from progressing.

THE PRICE OF EATING REFINED SUGARS

All differences aside, a big question remains for both allopathic and naturopathic doctors. Even if only 2% of people self-reporting symptoms can be diagnosed allopathically, that's still triple the number of people reporting symptoms just 60 years ago. Most of that dramatic increase has been in North America, some parts of Europe, and Australia.

Why has there been such a surge in food intolerance in just six decades? And why mostly in industrial nations?

There are numerous theories, but from a naturopathic perspective they all relate to the over-processing and manipulation of our food supply. Or to put it another way, the problems all begin in our intestines, the largest organ in the immune system.

Our bodies evolved over millions of years in relationship to the natural foods in our environment. We ate natural sugars embedded in complex carbohydrates. This ensured we had enough fibre in our diets. Fibre is important. It helps food move smoothly through the digestive tract. The goal of digestion is for food to be broken down enough in the mouth and stomach that by the time it reaches the intestines, the mucosa (intestinal lining) can do its job. Its job is to extract nutrients, transfer them into the blood to be distributed around the body, and eliminate waste products.

When we eat too many simple carbohydrates, food can move through the upper parts of the digestive system too quickly and then, when it reaches the lower parts, it can get backed up in the intestines, where it can literally sit and rot. Think about a compost heap: if it's decomposing properly, on a cold night, you should be able to see warm gas rising off of it. Rotting simple carbohydrates in your intestines generate gas too, which can make you feel bloated and cause cramping.

This also creates the perfect environment for certain types of bacteria to thrive. Don't get me wrong; I'm a big fan of bacteria. There are thousands of strains of bacteria in our bodies that are essential to helping food digest and fortifying the immune system. But if the environment in the intestines becomes unbalanced due to a backup of simple carbohydrates sitting there and rotting, it can cultivate the wrong kind of bacteria and even organisms like Candida Albicans. The wrong kind of organisms can throw off your body's micro flora balance, which is a big problem. That balance helps the body to:

- Defend itself against invading bacteria that could cause infection.
- Break down food so it can extract nutrients and transport them through the body.
- Maintain the health of the mucosa, which separates the waste in the bowels from the vital organs in the abdominal cavity.

63

- Maintain a healthy immune response

THE PRICE OF EATING HYDROGENATED FATS

We pay a price for eating refined sugars. Then we add hydrogenated fats. Trans-fats mixed with refined sugars make some of the most mouth-watering treats on the market, but remember that, at a molecular level, trans-fats are more like plastics than essential fats. Our bodies didn't evolve to digest plastics. Think about a compost heap again. If you put a hunk of plastic in the middle of it, it won't decompose along with everything else. It will decompose over a much longer time, but as it does, it won't release nutrients, but toxins.

The gut mucosa can't break down plastics any better than a compost heap can. The best thing your body can do with trans-fats is eliminate them, but if your digestive system is sluggish because of refined sugar, those trans-fats are likely to just sit in the intestines with all the other partially digested food, generating gas, cultivating the wrong type of bacteria, creating bacterial imbalance in your body, and possibly releasing toxins.

What's even worse about trans-fats is that they displace essential fatty acids (EFA); that is, they take up the space for the essential fats your body needs. In Chapter 4, I talked about the detrimental impacts of trans-fats, but I didn't list any of the positive roles EFA play in your body. Whole books have been written about the importance of EFA to overall health, but specifically in terms of avoiding food intolerances, EFAs:

- Control inflammatory processes: they help the body know when to trigger inflammation to expel an invader, and when to stop it.
- Keep skin strong, yet supple: the skin is the immune system's first line of defense against invaders, so allowing skin to break down is like allowing a breach in your defenses.
- Lubricate the digestive system: like fibre, lubrication keeps food moving through the digestive tract rather than getting backed up and sitting in the intestines.
- Sustain the health of the mucosa: this is crucial to helping your body absorb nutrients from food, secrete waste from your body,

and maintain a selectively permeable barrier that allows nutrients to flow out into the blood but keeps undigested food and waste in the intestines, where it belongs.

LEAKY GUT SYNDROME

When food slows down in the intestines and starts rotting, you can develop leaky gut syndrome, which allopathic doctors call hyperpermeability of the intestinal membrane. Leaky gut syndrome occurs when the intestinal mucosa is damaged, compromising its ability to protect your internal environment, and allowing bacteria, toxins, undigested food particles, and waste to "leak" out of the intestines and into the blood.

"This triggers an autoimmune reaction, which can lead to gastrointestinal problems such as abdominal bloating, excessive gas and cramps, fatigue, food sensitivities, joint pain, skin rashes, and autoimmunity," says Dr. Andrew Weil, a well-known MD who specializes in integrated medicine.* Leaky gut syndrome isn't well recognized by family physicians. Gastroenterologists (allopathic doctors who specialize in the gastrointestinal system) are starting to recognize it, but remain puzzled by it. However, what puzzles me most is their surprise when patients "resort" to alternative practitioners. Here's the way one article on *WebMD* described the problem, from an allopathic perspective:

> *Leaky gut symptoms aren't unique. They're shared by other problems, too. And tests often fail to uncover a definite cause of the problem. That can leave people without a diagnosis and, therefore, untreated.*
>
> *It's crucial . . . to find a doctor who will take time with you and take your concerns seriously.*

"You may have leaky gut and we may be able to treat what causes it," says gastroenterologist Donald Kirby, MD, director of the Center for Human Nutrition at the Cleveland Clinic. "If you have something going on, it is incumbent upon the medical community to listen to you," says Kirby.

---

* "What is Leaky Gut?" by Dr. Andrew Weil, *Weil*, http://www.drweil.com/drw/u/QAA361058/what-is-leaky-gut.html.

Unfortunately, "not all doctors make the effort to get at the root of the problem, and that's what frequently sends patients to alternative practitioners," says Linda A. Lee, MD, a gastroenterologist and director of the Johns Hopkins Integrative Medicine and Digestive Center

"Often, the reason they have resorted to alternative medicine is because of what they have been told and how they have been treated by other practitioners . . . We need to listen."[†]

Well, yes, listen – and perhaps not only to patients but to qualified members of other recognized health disciplines. I can't speak for all my colleagues, but I'd be happy to share my knowledge with gastroenterologists in the interests of patient health.

I might start by sharing the naturopathic perspective that food intolerance exists on a spectrum. We may not always be able to intervene to prevent it from progressing to a more severe and dangerous Ig-mediated response, but sometimes we can. And if we can prevent illness, isn't that better than waiting for it to develop enough so we can use differential diagnosis to name it? Why do we have to name a problem before we treat it? Why not believe the patient and treat the symptoms?

OTHER FACTORS IN FOOD INTOLERANCES

We can find support for the naturopathic view that food intolerances progress from sensitivity to allergy by looking at what's happening with food intolerance in different parts of the world. While wheat gluten is a big problem in North America, rice is a bigger problem in South East Asia, and sesame seeds in the Middle East. The allopathic view of food intolerances doesn't explain these regional variations. The only thing that explains them is that they develop partly because of over-exposure, which supports the naturopathic perspective that intolerance occurs on a spectrum.

But, over-exposure can't be the only factor. People have been eating the same things for thousands of years without developing intolerances. We can only understand the explosion in food intolerances since World War II by understanding that it's no

[†] "Leaky Gut Syndrome: What Is It?" by Matt McMillen, *WebMD*, http://www.webmd.com/digestive-disorders/features/leaky-gut-syndrome.

coincidence that it happened at the same time as we shifted to mass-producing foods, over-processing them to extend shelf life, and then using chemicals to mimic the flavour and colour we've stripped out, all based on the principles behind the 3 Ps.

There have been other factors, as well, of course. For example:

- There's the "hygiene hypothesis," which suggests we've become too clean, decreasing our contact with the many bacteria we need to sustain intestinal health.
- Increased rates of Caesarean birth could be contributing. Babies born vaginally pick up bacteria in the birth canal that they need to colonize their intestines, while babies born by C-section pick up unhealthy bacteria from the hospital environment.
- Several studies have shown breastfeeding protects babies from developing food allergies, especially if it's continued through at least the first six months of life, when the baby's immune system has matured somewhat. So, a decrease in breastfeeding could be a factor in food intolerances.
- It's also likely chemical sensitivity is playing a role in increasing rates of food intolerance, by sensitizing and weakening our "neurovascular, endocrine, gastrointestinal, respiratory (including ear, nose, and throat), genitourinary, musculoskeletal, and dermal systems."[‡]

It's probably no coincidence that most of the factors contributing to food intolerance are related in some way to the digestive tract. As I've said, the intestines play a key role in the immune system and therefore also a key role in food intolerance.

FOOD INTOLERANCES AND THE 3 PS

An interesting twist is occurring in the global food industry right now. With millions of people seeking gluten-free, dairy-free, and nut-free foods, the same industry that played a key role in creating the problem of food intolerance is making significant profit from it. A report from Agriculture and Agri-Foods Canada described the

‡ "Chemical Hypersensitivity and the Allergic Response," *Ear, Nose, and Throat Journal,* Volume 67, Issue 1, Jan 1988, http://www.aehf.com/articles/article36.html.

growing incidence of food intolerances as a positive development from a marketing perspective because it shows the market will be profitable for a long time.

It's tempting to leap from there to a conspiracy theory blaming the food industry for food intolerances, but blame is an easy way to dodge personal responsibility. We've created our own food intolerances by buying and eating processed foods, and now we very much need products for people who have developed food intolerances.

At the same time as we're using those products to cope with our own or our children's food intolerances, let's remain aware of our need to take responsibility for our own health from now on, and to teach our children to do the same. Let's skip the blame, understand the role the 3 Ps play in health, and start making better choices than we've made in the past. One way we can do that is by understanding the role stress plays in health. That's what I'll discuss in the next chapter.

CHAPTER 6:
HOW DID STRESS TAKE OVER OUR LIVES?

I remember a classic case of a patient who'd become very ill with digestive problems. He was 30 years old, about 5'10", and 150 pounds – fairly thin. He'd been having abdominal symptoms for some time. His appetite was poor, he couldn't keep food down, and he had frequent, loose, bloody stools.

His gastroenterologist had told him it was irritable bowel syndrome (IBS), bordering on colitis. When he came to his first appointment with me, he had a little plastic bag of pill bottles. He had drugs to slow his bowels down, reduce the inflammation, and heal the tearing – a different drug for each sign and symptom.

"I don't like taking all these pills, he said, and I don't like the side effects. My specialist says if I stop taking them my bowels could ulcerate and then she'd have to surgically remove a section of my colon. But there has to be another way. This can't be it for the rest of my life."

I started taking his history. One of my questions was when he was most likely to have bowel movements.

"Usually right before I go to school," he said.

It's common for IBS patients to have an attack of diarrhea right before school or work. That told me what questions I should ask next.

"How would you describe your temperament?" I asked. "Do you sleep well? Do you bite your nails or have any repetitive behaviours? Do you have reflux or headaches?"

He said he'd been a high-strung child who'd get upset easily and then have to run to the bathroom. Lately he hadn't been sleeping well. He was having issues at school, which were stressful because he was trying to get into law school. A friend had suggested his problems might be related to food intolerances, so he thought he'd try a naturopathic doctor.

"I can check for food intolerances," I said. "But I doubt they're the underlying cause of your problems."

Sure enough, I found a few problem foods, and he got them out of his diet. He felt a little better, but not as well as he'd hoped, so I suggested we check his cortisol levels.

"What is cortisol and what does it have to do with my bowels?" He asked.

"The digestive tract is like a disassembly line," I explained. "As food goes through, your digestive system takes it apart piece by piece. Cortisol is a hormone that plays an important role in the stress response. When you're under a lot of stress, your cortisol levels increase. That speeds up your whole system – heart rate, breathing, digestion, everything. Food moves through your gastrointestinal tract too quickly and reaches your intestines without being properly digested. That's where the problems start. The way to get them under control is to reduce and manage your stress levels."

Although this young man had a few food intolerances, they weren't the main source of his problems. Stress was. He needed to continue taking drugs to manage his symptoms in the short term, but I also gave him supplements to heal his gut lining, and he found ways to reduce and manage his stress. It took close to a year, but he was finally able to get off the medications and get on with his life.

STRESS: A CASCADE OF EFFECTS

In balanced amounts, stress is healthy. Stress provides a burst of energy and sharpens the mind. It can improve heart function and strengthen the immune system. Stress can help you get things done quickly and well, such as meeting a deadline. Stress can protect against Alzheimer's by keeping brain cells agile, and help your body recover more quickly from surgery. One study found that "children of mothers who had higher levels of the stress hormone cortisol during pregnancy were developmentally ahead of those of women with lower levels."[*]

When stress becomes continuous and constantly floods your body with its powerful hormones, you begin to feel its negative effects. IBS is a common outcome of stress, because stress often strikes the digestive system first, but also I've treated countless patients with eczema, arthritis, migraines, asthma, or food intolerances only to find that these issues were really symptoms of underlying stress.

I'm confused. How can stress be both healthy and unhealthy?

Think of the stress response as a cascade of effects on the body. A cascade of water over rocks can be a beautiful waterfall, unless it becomes a flood, and then it can destroy anything in its path. The cascade of stress effects has its source in the adrenal gland. We don't understand the adrenal gland well, but I believe allopathic medicine underestimates its importance, as well as the role adrenal hormones play in illness. The adrenal gland produces numerous hormones. When stress begins, the adrenal gland releases a hormone called cortisol, which triggers the fight-or-flight response.

THE EVOLUTION OF THE STRESS RESPONSE

The stress response evolved over millions of years to give people a burst of speed, strength, and precision right when they needed it. Today, however, you're rarely running away from a threat or hunting for your dinner. You're more likely stressed from sitting in traffic or meeting a deadline. Yet your body is still in a state of stimulation: your blood pressure rises, your heart rate increases, your breathing quickens, your hair stands on end, and your pupils dilate. You might be in that state for a long time, which means the cortisol will stay in your body for a long time, unless you do something to get rid of it, like go for a workout.

But that's not always possible, and the same cortisol that helps you meet that deadline can seriously damage your body if it remains at high levels for a long time. Being "sick to your stomach" in

---

[*] "Can Stress Actually Be Good For You?" *NBCNews.com*, http://www.nbcnews.com/id/15818153/ns/health-mental_health/t/can-stress-actually-be-good-you/#.U5ZIByjb4TF

a stressful situation is one symptom of high cortisol. Cortisol stimulates your intestinal nerves, causing faster motility, loose stools, cramps, and bloating, which are all symptoms of IBS. It also stimulates release of stomach acid, which can give you acid reflux.

Cortisol can also cause fatigue. If your cortisol level is out of control, you can feel like you've just run a marathon after a walk to the corner store. And then there's muscle tension. Cortisol tenses your muscles and elevates your blood pressure, but if that keeps up you can end up with debilitating headaches and back pain for days on end. Cortisol can make you feel nervous and anxious, causing insomnia. It can even irritate nerve endings in your skin, triggering release of oils that cause acne, or histamines that cause eczema.

All these symptoms are typical of an excessive adrenal response. If they happen occasionally, there will probably be no harm done. But when stress occurs repeatedly and for extended periods of time, serious problems can set in, including physical issues, like IBS, and mental wellness issues, such as depression and anxiety.

Perhaps the biggest problem with stress-related illness is that it can build for years, but you might not see it coming because the symptoms seem to creep up slowly and then hit all at once. The reason you don't notice is that another adrenal hormone, called DHEA, counteracts cortisol's effects, bringing your heart rate and breathing back to normal. It restores balance to your system.

So if DHEA restores balance, what's the problem?

You've heard the expression "the last straw." As the saying goes, you can keep adding one piece of straw after another to a camel's back, but even though each piece weighs almost nothing, at some point you'll add one straw too many and it will break the camel's back.

Stress works the same way. You think you're coping, but one day you add that last straw, and your continuing high levels of cortisol finally deplete your adrenal gland's ability to release DHEA. Your body becomes unable to cope, and you begin to experience more complex and enduring symptoms.

THE INSULIN RESPONSE

One enduring symptom of stress is related to blood sugar and insulin levels. Insulin is a hormone that regulates blood sugar and metabolism. High blood sugar can cause weight gain, while low blood sugar can cause you to shake, sweat, and become disoriented, or even lose consciousness. The right amount of insulin prevents blood sugar from rising too high or falling too low.

However, as I said in chapter 4, when cortisol levels are high, insulin sensitivity starts to drop. In this case, insulin sensitivity decreases as part of the fight-or-flight response: sugar provides energy when you need to fight or run away, so reduced insulin sensitivity makes more sugar available to your body when you need it. But if your cortisol stays high and your insulin sensitivity stays low, your blood sugar levels can become unstable. Your body can become accustomed to high blood sugar, causing you to feel constantly hungry and crave sugar.

And sugar is addictive!

Exactly! Say you're feeling stressed about studying for exams. You crave sugar, reach for a chocolate bar, and get a burst of endorphins. But if you do that often, it can become a habit, and even an addiction. It can cause you to gain weight, increase your risk of diabetes, increase your levels of bad cholesterol, and trigger high blood pressure. Suddenly, without thinking it would ever happen to you, you're one of those people struggling to manage diabetes, fight heart disease, or overcome cancer. A lot of people think stress is simply a state of mind, but the connection between stress and chronic disease aptly illustrates something we call the mind-body connection.

What's the mind-body connection?

I'll talk about it in Chapter 10, but for now knowing your mind and body work together might help you understand that so-called mental health issues, such as anxiety and depression, are closely related to physical health. When your adrenal gland is stressed, it doesn't only trigger what you might think of as physical symptoms. It also affects your body's ability to produce hormones that mediate your mood. If your adrenal gland becomes too taxed, you can experience depression. If your cortisol levels are always high, you can have anxiety attacks. If you're seeking solace in food, you could develop an eating disorder.

HOW DID WE GET HERE FROM THERE?

Let's take a step back and review. Just 300 years ago, the Industrial Revolution initiated dramatic changes in farming and manufacturing. It began a massive movement of the population from subsistence farms to crowded cities. Over the next 150 years, the ideas behind the concept I call the 3 Ps began to slowly take hold. People hailed each new advance in technology or industry without thinking about long-term consequences.

Even 60 years ago, one-third of the North American population lived on farms. Life moved at a slower pace. World War II brought incredible advances in agricultural technology, prescription medicines, and mass production of food. After the war, people were ready for peace and prosperity. The advent of television put enviable lifestyles in everyone's living room. The advertising industry grew, creating demand for products and lifestyles. The food industry grew, appealing to people who were working longer hours to pay for those lifestyles. The pharmaceutical industry grew, offering easy answers whenever anyone got sick.

Maybe if the changes had happened over just a few short years, some people would have made the connections and said, "Stop! Slow down! It's all happening too fast. We're getting too stressed. We're eating the wrong foods. We're getting sick and then trying to fix it with drugs. We're losing control of our health and we have to take it back." But the changes happened over a long enough time, and most people were so busy and stressed, that few people connected the rapid changes around them with the rapidly rising rates of chronic diseases like diabetes, heart disease, arthritis, and cancer.

The good news is that we can take back control of our lives and our health. Remember the story at the start of Chapter 5 about the 60-year-old woman with rheumatoid arthritis? I left off when she achieved some improvement as a result of identifying food intolerances, but that's not where her story ended. To find out her very happy ending, read Chapter 7 and learn about toxic load.

CHAPTER 7:
HOW HAS TOXIC LOAD BECOME A HEALTH ISSUE?

As you may recall, the patient I described at the beginning of chapter 5 was a 60-year-old woman with rheumatoid arthritis. After achieving a 15% improvement in her symptoms by addressing food intolerances, she agreed to cortisol testing to evaluate how her body was coping with stress. She'd already said that, as the eldest in a large family, she'd often been responsible for her younger siblings, and now she was taking care of her mother.

"I've just never had time in my life to focus on myself," she said. "But now, I have time. And I'm motivated."

"In that case," I said. "I suggest we proceed with a four-point cortisol test to evaluate how your body is handling stress."

The test showed her morning cortisol level at the low end of normal, while her night-time cortisol was quite high. Clearly, she was not sleeping well because of stress and was therefore not waking up feeling rested and energized. I recommended some supplements to support her adrenal glands and increase her morning cortisol, and others to decrease her night-time cortisol levels.

"I can't believe how much better I'm sleeping already," she said on a subsequent visit. "I have so much more energy during the day. And my muscles seem to be loosening up, finally, after years of feeling stiff and sore all the time. "

However, all was not well yet. Although her arthritis symptoms were, by now, about 50% better, and sleeping better had improved her outlook in general, she was still suffering from joint inflammation.

"What else could it be?" She asked.

"I'm wondering about heavy metal toxicity," I said.

"Where would that be coming from?" She asked.

"Life in the twenty-first century," I said. "Although we've smartened up about lead pipes and lead in paints, there's still a lot residual lead in our environment, and in some products we import from countries without the same regulations we have here. And it's impossible to eat fish or seafood without absorbing some mercury. Some people eliminate these toxins from their bodies better than others."

Blood tests for heavy metals revealed extremely high levels of lead and mercury. I started her on a comprehensive treatment protocol, and soon her joint inflammation began to lessen. Within a year, she was 90% free of arthritis symptoms. With such dramatic progress, there was no need to pursue testing further, so we continued with treatment to maintain her health status, including dietary improvements and an exercise routine.

The best part of the story came a few months later. This now 61-year-old woman who had limped into my office a year earlier with swollen joints and a cane, but full of motivation to make the most of what life still had to offer, pursued the dream she'd been holding onto for decades: she bought a ticket, got on a plane, and went backpacking through Europe.

TOXINS: WHEN ORGANIC IS NOT A GOOD THING

From a naturopathic perspective, there are two types of toxins: inorganics, which are naturally occurring heavy metals, sometimes also called elementals; and organics, which are synthetic toxins like preservatives, pesticides, and chemicals in cleaning products, personal hygiene products, and cosmetics.

There are thousands of organic toxins, making it virtually impossible to test for all of them. In the book *Slow Death by Rubber Duck,* the authors look at some of the most common organic toxins in our daily environment, and the seemingly innocuous places they may lurk. The toxins they list include:

- Phthalates: which makes plastic strong yet flexible. Phthalates have been linked with reproductive and developmental problems and issues with the endocrine system (a collection of glands that secrete hormones transported to virtually every organ in the body).

- Perflourinated chemicals (PFCs): which are commonly found in non-stick coatings like Teflon pans and microwave popcorn bags, and sprayed onto fabrics and carpets to make them stain resistant. PFCs have been linked with many types of cancer, as well as developmental problems in children.
- Brominated flame retardants (PBDEs): which are soaked into fabrics to make babies' sleepers and other children's clothing, as well as electronics and upholstery. These can interfere with children's hormonal, reproductive, thyroid, metabolic, and neurological development.
- Triclosan: an antibacterial chemical used in products ranging from soap-free hand disinfectants to sports socks to satisfy our almost pathological fear of germs. It has been associated with immune system and endocrine system dysfunction.
- Bisphenol-A (BP-A): used in the linings of metal cans to prevent oxidation, as well as baby bottles, plastic storage containers, and dental sealants. It has been linked with problems in the endocrine system.

This list does not include all the pesticides sprayed on our foods, pollutants from burning fossil fuels, and so on, but rather those we often overlook because we can't imagine why children's toys, clothing, or baby bottles would include things harmful to their development – or how electronics or furniture could emit toxic gases into our homes.

Many chemicals are harmful because they accumulate in fatty tissues, so we don't eliminate them through our sweat or urine. This makes it wise to try to avoid them as much as possible. For example, we can use tempered glass baby bottles and food storage containers rather than plastic ones, and cook with pots and pans that are not Teflon coated. We can make popcorn the old-fashioned way, wear clothing made from natural, untreated fibres, and use cleaning products made from natural products. We can also worry a little less about disinfecting everything around us, keeping in mind that our obsession with killing bacteria could also be contributing to a lack of intestinal bacteria, which could contribute to food intolerances.

I'll talk more about avoiding organic toxins in Chapters 23 and 25. However, as background information about them is not one of my areas of expertise, I won't delve into them any further here. If I suspected a patient's problems originated with organic toxins, I'd refer him to someone with the appropriate knowledge and skills.

TOXINS: THE INORGANIC KIND

When I test for toxic load, I focus on inorganic toxins, which include heavy metals and some metalloids (chemicals that are somewhere between metals and non-metals). Unlike a confusing array of organic toxins, inorganics are easy to identify and measure. Like organics, inorganics can accumulate over time in tissues, making it difficult for us to eliminate them from our bodies. The primary health concern is their effect on brain chemistry. This could play a role in developing Alzheimer's disease, as well digestive issues, heart disease, and various cancers, among other things.

Toxic exposure is of particular concern in children, because their gastrointestinal function has not yet matured. Toxins can leach out of their intestines into their blood and cross the blood-brain barrier, which is more permeable in children than adults. Children may also absorb arsenic, a metalloid, by inhaling second-hand tobacco smoke.

Inorganic toxins are also of special concern in pregnant women because metals that have been absorbed into bone tissues may leach into the blood stream and cross the placental barrier, where they can cause a range of developmental issues, and sometimes birth defects. The most likely cause is chronic, low-level exposure, building up in our bodies over a long period of time and contributing to degenerative health issues as we age.

Inorganic toxins cause damage in two ways: through oxidative damage, and by mimicking essential nutrients. Oxidation is a natural process of decomposition. When fruit rots or a piece of metal rusts, it's oxidizing. Oxidation is beneficial in the body because it helps eliminate pathogens, such as bacteria or viruses, but too much oxidation can damage essential systems.

A number of things can cause excessive oxidative reactions, including refined sugars, trans-fats, cigarette smoke, chemicals, and inorganic toxins. Oxidative stress is believed to contribute to cancer, heart disease, Parkinson's disease, and Alzheimer's disease, among other conditions that are often considered inevitable aspects of aging.

Many inorganic toxins can also mimic the action of nutrients essential to our health in trace amounts; in essence, they "fool" cells into absorbing them instead of absorbing the real nutrients. For example, cadmium can compete with proteins, enzymes, and zinc for absorption into cells, lead can also displace calcium, and thallium can mimic potassium in nerves and the cardiovascular system. So, as well as causing oxidative damage, inorganic toxins can deprive cells of essential nutrients.

There's a difference between acute toxicity caused by sudden, significant exposure to a toxin, and a slow build-up of toxins over time as a result of chronic low-level exposure. Allopathic doctors consider heavy metal toxicity rare because allopathic research has not yet conclusively demonstrated that chronic build-up of toxins does not need to reach acute levels to cause powerful negative reactions. This is the type of toxicity we see most often in naturopathic medicine.

CHRONIC MERCURY AND LEAD TOXICITY

Mercury and lead are the biggest areas of concern in my practice. Mercury is one of the oldest poisons known to humans, and one of the most toxic. In the past, despite its known toxic effects, mercury was used in large amounts for many purposes. In modern times, it's rarely present in large enough amounts to cause extensive damage, but in small amounts it's used for dozens of purposes in everyday life.

Mercury has been used in tilt switches, which make the light go on when you open your freezer or the trunk of your car; in fluorescent and neon lights; in many types of thermometers, barometers, and manometers; in batteries; combined with other metals, like silver, to create an amalgam, such as for dental fillings; as a fungicide in bathroom, kitchen, and hospital paints; as a fungicide on potatoes, among other crops; and as a preservative in vaccines.

Many of these uses have been banned in industrial nations, but mercury never disappears, so some older products are still in use and products dumped in landfills continue to leach mercury into the environment. As well, in nations that don't regulate burning coal for fuel, smokestacks belch mercury into the air much as they did during the Industrial Revolution. Mercury then makes its way around the world, contaminating many species of fish and seafood and creating a dilemma: fish contains EFA, which are vital to health, but eating too much fish can drive blood mercury beyond safe levels.

The Life Extension Foundation lists a wide range of health problems caused by mercury:

> *...mercury can cause widespread toxicity and symptoms in several organ systems: nervous system (eg, personality changes, tremors, memory deficits, loss of coordination); cardiovascular system (eg, increased risk of arterial obstruction, hypertension, stroke, atherosclerosis, heart attacks, and increased inflammation); GI tract (eg, nausea, diarrhea, ulceration); and kidneys (failure). Mercury may also accumulate in the thyroid and increase the risk of autoimmune disorders, and may cause contact dermatitis.*[*]

Children can suffer from cognitive deficits and impaired motor skills even with very low levels of mercury in their blood. However, in my practice, my concern is more with older patients and the link between mercury contamination and degenerative neurological disorders such as Alzheimer's and Parkinson's. Although the scientific research remains inconclusive, I've seen too many cases of low-level heavy metal contamination, like that of the woman with arthritis, to dismiss them all as anecdotal, and therefore invalid.

Lead exposure can come from a variety of sources. Factory workers from plants that manufacture lead-containing products – ranging from batteries to radiation shields for X-ray technicians – can inhale lead dust, as well as bringing it home on their clothing, unwittingly exposing their children to it. In the past, lead was often

---

[*] "Heavy Metal Detoxification," *Life Extension Foundation for Longer Life,*
http://www.lef.org/protocols/health_concerns/heavy_metal_detoxification_02.htm.

used to give paint its vibrant colours, and it continues to hang around in older homes, where chipped paint around windows turns to dust and is absorbed through the skin.

Although industrial nations have banned lead in paint, factories in developing nations still make children's toys and furniture with lead-containing paints. Though industrial nations banned lead-containing gas many years ago, the ground beneath decommissioned gas stations may still be contaminated and leaching lead into groundwater. Kohl, an ancient cosmetic from the Middle East, also contains lead. The possible sources of low-level lead contamination are many, and often surprising.

Because lead mimics calcium, the human body tends to store lead in bones. It can remain there for decades, until fractures, pregnancy, or age-related bone loss releases it. Sometimes it will be eliminated through feces or urine, but it may also enter the blood and travel to organs throughout the body. Chronic low-level lead exposure can cause gastrointestinal issues, hypertension, and kidney dysfunction. As levels increase, it may disrupt thyroid and reproductive hormones, and interfere with brain function. Low-level lead exposure in children can cause a range of developmental disorders.

While mercury and lead are the most common causes of toxicity I see, you should be aware of several other inorganic toxins, such as cadmium, arsenic, and aluminum. Again, some of these pop up in unlikely places. Aluminum, for example, is not only absorbed into our foods from cookware, but is also an ingredient in deodorant and an adjuvant (to boost effectiveness) in many vaccines.

Chemotherapy makes wise use of heavy metals to kill cancer cells, which is not easy. If you've survived cancer, you may be very grateful for this, and I would never discourage anyone from receiving life-saving treatments, but once you're well again, remember that some of the toxins may linger in your body causing health issues, called late effects. These can include hormonal problems, bone loss, joint pain, and cognitive deficits, among other problems. Naturopathic detoxification protocols may help.

NOT TO BE DISMISSED

In some ways, awareness of problems with inorganic toxins is better now than historically because there are regulations, at least in the industrial world, against causing acute exposure. But in other ways, inorganic toxins are more problematic now than ever because they're present at low levels in so many places we wouldn't suspect.

Allopathic doctors and medical researchers tend to dismiss the idea that low-level exposure over long periods of time can lead to toxic build-up. This is no one's fault. Because it takes place over a long period of time, it's difficult for researchers to establish a pattern of cause and effect, and that pattern is crucial to allopathic diagnosis and treatment.

But I've seen many patients whose allopathic doctors have said their symptoms were aspects of chronic degenerative diseases and could only be managed with drugs. Yet, like the woman who went backpacking through Europe, they've responded well to detoxification protocols. I've also seen many patients who have been told their symptoms are inevitable facets of aging for which there are no treatments. I'll talk about managing the aging process in the next chapter.

CHAPTER 8:
CAN WE CONTROL THE AGING PROCESS?

Some years ago, a man in his sixties came into the clinic. He was retired, but during his working life he'd been very successful in business, no doubt because of his aggressive, competitive nature. Since retiring, he'd been teaching at business school, and sharing a lifetime of knowledge had kept him feeling young and vigorous. But he'd recently felt he was losing his drive.

"I've played tennis all my life," he said. "And I play to win. But over the last year, I've lost my competitive edge. My partner is beating me so often it isn't fun for either of us anymore. And I'm thinking of giving up teaching because I just don't think I have anything left to give the students."

"What about other areas of your life?" I asked. "How are things at home, with your wife?"

"You mean my libido?" He asked. "Almost non-existent. I'm not sure she even finds me attractive anymore."

"Have you spoken to your family doctor about this?" I asked.

"He said I was just getting older and maybe I should learn to sit back and enjoy life more," he said.

"What do you think about that?" I asked.

"I was enjoying life before," he said.

This struck me as a classic problem with age management. There were no body composition issues, no food intolerances, and if anything, he missed having stress in his life. His allopathic doctor had ruled out disease, and he showed no symptoms of toxic load. All that remained was wellness testing.

I tested his androgen, testosterone, and DHEA levels (DHEA is converted into testosterone), as well as several other hormones and proteins that regulate body processes and provide that zest for life he was missing. He'd been concerned about a family history of heart disease, so I tested his blood levels of homocysteine and CRP,* both of which can be risk factors for heart disease.

Sure enough, his androgen, testosterone, and DHEA were low, which explained his lack of energy, low libido, and loss of competitive drive. I prescribed supplements to bring his hormone levels back up again and reduce his homocysteine and CRP levels.

"So how's it going?" I asked when he returned to the clinic several weeks later.

"I've got my tennis game back!" He said. "And let's just say I was wrong in thinking my wife no longer found me attractive."

His naturally aggressive and competitive nature had returned and his personal life was back on track. He'd been at risk not only of having an uneventful retirement, but of slipping into depression because he'd lost his sense of the man he'd been all his life. With a few supplements, he was able to get that back.

LOOKING YOUNG VS. FEELING GOOD

Have you ever met a person and thought they were a few years older than you, and then found out they're actually the same age as you, or a little younger?

Yes – usually after I've said something to offend them about their age!

In those cases, it's likely that a few tests to measure what I call markers of aging and wellness would show the person's body performing as if they were a few years older than they are.

Are you talking about those infomercials that claim to reverse the aging process?

No! We're all aging from the moment we're born. Outside of getting to 39 and counting your birthdays backward, you can't reverse the aging process. The thing to remember about TV advertising is that it costs a lot of money. So whether an ad is selling an anti-aging product or a convenience food, you know right away the first priority is profit.

---

* I'll define these later in this chapter.

Those infomercials often use terms like "free radicals" and "antioxidants," which sound very scientific. Didn't you use those terms in the last chapter?

Ads for so-called anti-aging products often use legitimate scientific terminology to sell products they claim will make you look younger. But the goal of aging well is not to look young; it's to be healthy. If you're healthy, you will look good. Products sold from an anti-aging angle take advantage of your fear of aging, but that fear comes from the belief that age and illness are the same.

That's another aspect of our attitude about doing things that are terrible for our health until illness arises, and then taking pills to make it go away. The consequence of living that way is suffering the cumulative effects that eventually result in chronic degenerative disease. We've become so accustomed to this idea that we now simply accept that aging means being sick, and looking unhealthy. I've seen 90-year-olds who still look vibrant and full of life, because they are. I've also seen 50-year-olds who look like they're heading for an early grave.

Aging is a process we all go through. The levels of certain hormones and proteins in our bodies change as we age; for example, women's levels of estrogen and men's testosterone levels decrease with age. This is a normal and natural part of aging. However, in some people, these markers of age change earlier in life than would be considered normal. The result is that a patient's body ages faster biologically than chronologically. A variety of factors may have influenced this accelerated aging process. These factors might include:

- Genetic predisposition
- Poor dietary habits
- Lack of exercise
- Weight gain
- Physical or emotional trauma
- Use of alcohol, tobacco, or caffeine
- Use of OTC or prescription drugs
- Recreational use of illegal drugs
- Exposure to organic toxins (such as pesticides and air pollutants)

- Exposure to inorganic toxins (heavy metals and metalloids)

If you look at the above list, you'll see that many of the factors contributing to early aging are things we've already discussed. You have no control over your genetic predisposition, but every other item on the list is within your control. But, in our culture, particularly in the last 70 years, we have lost control over simple aspects of health like body composition (including diet and exercise), food intolerances, stress levels, and toxic load. An accelerated aging process can be a culmination of all the aspects of life in the twenty-first century that have spiralled out of our control.

Patients whose bodies are showing signs of premature aging may be at risk for developing one or more of the chronic diseases we've been discussing. Although my focus in this book is primarily on diabetes, heart disease, arthritis, and cancer, premature aging can also increase your risk for developing Alzheimer's or Parkinson's disease, osteoporosis, cataracts, glaucoma, or hearing loss.

These conditions do not develop overnight, but over years. Almost everyone who develops any of these conditions have experienced some of these symptoms during that time. But, in our fast-paced culture with its focus on working long hours, eating junk foods, and accumulating possessions, most of us have not developed the good habit of listening to our bodies' attempts to communicate with us. We notice symptoms, but ignore them until they are so pronounced we can no longer deny them. And then we go to an allopathic doctor seeking a diagnosis, a prescription, and even surgery to make symptoms go away so we can go on with our lives as usual!

STRESS AND AGING

One of the key factors that can make us age prematurely is stress. If you look at pictures of President Bill Clinton at age 47, when he began his eight years in the White House, and then again eight years later, you'll see a man who went from a little salt and pepper in his hair to snowy white hair. Now do the same for President Barack Obama. He was also 47 when first elected. Just four years later, the differences in his face and hair were remarkable.

Research into stress and aging shows that stress does, in effect, wear our bodies down. An article in *Psychology Today* explained that stress-related aging is caused by three things: oxidation, glycation, and diminishing telomeres. As I've said, oxidation is a process of decomposition, and it's been linked with heart disease, Alzheimer's, arthritis, and many other diseases we associate with aging. Glycation occurs through a complicated process during glucose (sugar) metabolism, and it impairs circulation, stiffens skin, and causes body tissues to malfunction. Telomeres, which are found at the ends of our chromosomes, decrease with age, but researchers are exploring how anxiety and stress speed up this natural process, leading to an increase in cell death related to wrinkles, graying, and other signs of age.

None of these processes are things we can see or keep track of ourselves, but we can use several hormones and proteins as markers of aging. Research has provided the correct ranges for these markers depending on age and sex, and I use that to determine whether a patient's body is functioning at an older age than it should be. If it is, these markers can also help me predict if this patient is at increased risk for heart disease, diabetes, arthritis, or any other disease we associate with aging.

MARKERS OF AGE, PREDICTORS OF DISEASE

The following list describes the key measurable markers of age, and how I use them to predict susceptibility to chronic degenerative diseases:

- Fasting Insulin: the body uses insulin mainly to control blood sugar. Too much insulin means the body is having a hard time maintaining healthy blood sugar levels. Over time, this can cause a drop in insulin sensitivity, and then a drop in insulin levels, both of which can result in high blood sugar and diabetes. Insulin levels are a great way to predict diabetes risk and take steps to minimize risk.
- IGF-1 (Insulin-like Growth Factor): I test IGF-1 to assess overall degeneration of mind and body, and your body's healing potential—its ability to rejuvenate your health. IGF-1 is

important in preventing cellular breakdown, especially in muscle, cartilage, and brain tissue. If your IGF-1 is low, you may take longer to recover from injuries, which can be an indicator of accelerated aging.

- IGFBP-3 (Insulin-like Growth Factor Binding Protein): IGFBP-3 helps me assess growth hormone (GH) levels. A drop in GH may lead to weight gain, poor body composition, poor recovery from injury, and typical signs of aging in the hair, skin, and nails. Low IGFBP-3 may tell me you're suffering from malnutrition, and specifically low protein intake. High levels have been linked with an increased risk of heart disease, as well as prostate and breast cancers.
- SHBG (Sex Hormone Binding Globulin): this hormone regulates healthy estrogen and testosterone levels, and I test it to help assess those levels. As we age, our levels of these hormones gradually increase. Moreover, constant fluctuations in sex hormones can contribute to degenerative diseases, such as osteoarthritis, as well as ligament injury, and wrinkled or sagging skin.
- CRP (C- Reactive Protein): high levels of this protein can indicate inflammation in the body. Chronic inflammation can be a key sign of premature aging, and can lead to countless health problems, including heart disease, arthritis, cancer, diabetes, and dementia. Managing this protein level can help prevent many diseases often associated with aging.
- Homocysteine: homocysteine is an amino acid. One of the building blocks that make up proteins, we acquire it mostly by eating meat. High homocysteine is related to early development of heart and blood vessel disease. It is considered an independent risk factor for heart disease, which means that, even if no other factors indicate risk of heart disease, high homocysteine levels do.
- Estradiol, Progesterone and Testosterone (total versus free versus biologically available levels): monitoring and regulating sex hormones can help to maintain good health in several ways and slow down symptoms of menopause and andropause (male menopause).

- PSA (males): this is a protein produced by the prostate gland. This test is used to screen for and monitor prostate cancer. This is a good tool, but not a perfect one, because it can predict for the likelihood of developing prostate cancer, but it can't diagnose cancer, and it can't differentiate between slow-growing prostate tumors and very fast-growing, aggressive ones.
- Growth Hormone (GH): as we age, GH levels can drop sharply. This reduction plays a key role in aging, as the body becomes slower at repairing itself and recovering on a cellular level after illness or injury. Maintaining healthy levels of this hormone can slow the degenerative effects of aging.
- Albumin: this is an abundant protein in the body, and testing levels is a standard way to screen for many diseases. Low albumin levels can signify liver disease, kidney disease, and Crohn's disease. They can also indicate that a person is drinking too much alcohol, even if they are denying it.
- DHEA-S (Dehydroepiandrosterone): many health care practitioners call DHEA-S "the fountain of youth." Produced by the adrenal gland, levels of this hormone progressively decrease with age. In some body tissues, DHEA-S is converted into testosterone, so low DHEA-S may mean low testosterone. Low testosterone has been linked with many negative aspects of aging, such as muscle atrophy, decreased libido, reduced motivation, weight gain, and poor body composition.
- Free T3 (Triiodothyronine): this is a thyroid hormone. Low levels of thyroid hormones are linked with hypothyroidism (not enough thyroid activity) and high levels are linked hyperthyroidism (too much thyroid activity). Prompt treatment can restore levels to normal.

Although we can't directly control the levels of these markers in our bodies, there are other factors we can control, which in turn affect these levels. These factors are somewhat determined by genetics, but to a great extent they're controlled by lifestyle. Chronic illness doesn't have to be an inevitable part of aging. We can take steps to live life to the fullest for as long as possible.

DOING IT FOR OUR CHILDREN

Just as it is crucial to understanding our own responsibility in maintaining our health well into our senior years, so is it important to understand our responsibility to the next generation. Children are like little sponges. They soak up everything we say and do, and follow our example. More often than not, they live their lives very much as we have lived ours. So if we choose to ignore our health until we lose it, our children will likely do the same.

In the next chapter, I'll look at how we lost control of our children's health. This is the crux of the concept I call Generational Health First. When you take back control of your health, you teach your child by your example of how to live a healthy life, and they teach their children, who teach their children, and so on. I can't say it often enough: if we were all to start making generational health our first priority, within a few generations, we wouldn't need to think about it anymore. It would just be part of life.

CHAPTER 9:
HOW DID WE LOSE CONTROL OF OUR CHILDREN'S HEALTH?

One evening, a few summers ago, I got a call at home from my good friend, Mike, who contributed to this book. He has a little girl who was not quite two at the time, and she was sick with a very high fever. All parents worry when their children get sick, and a high fever can be particularly frightening.

"It's amazing how hot such a small child's body can get," he said. "She's lethargic, maybe even a little delirious. I want to make sure we're doing the right things."

"What are you doing?" I asked.

"Well, for one thing, I'm reminding myself that fever isn't a bad thing and I'm not going to the store to get acetaminophen." He said.

"That's a good start," I said. "What else?"

"We've got her in the bathroom, and we're sponging her down with cool water to keep her fever from climbing too high," he said. "And to make her more comfortable."

"That's good," I said. "What about dehydration?"

"We've got some cool water in a bottle mixed with a little bit of apple juice," he said.

"Is she able to suck on ice chips?" I asked.

"She's so out of it I'd be afraid she'd choke," he said.

"Then you're doing all the right things," I said.

Usually, when a small child spikes a high fever, the first thing parents do is reach for acetaminophen, which is sometimes sold under the brand name Tylenol, on the theory that if that doesn't bring the fever down, they're going to the hospital, but Mike knows that fever is not a bad thing, but a sign of healthy immune function.

Sure enough, by morning, the little girl's fever had come down. Her body had successfully fought off the virus.

"She's chattering and playing happily," Mike said when I spoke to him later that day. "The only problem is that neither my wife nor I got any sleep, but we still have to carry on with our day."

"There's nothing I can recommend for that," I said. "That's just one of the hazards of parenting!"

TAKE CONTROL OF YOUR CHILD'S HEALTH WITH INFORMATION

If you're a parent, you know how it feels to want to protect your child. But if you try to protect them too much, your goal of keeping them safe may backfire. If you keep them indoors all the time, they'll watch TV and play video games and their bodies won't grow strong. If you fill their schedules with activities that leave no time for unstructured play, they won't learn to be resourceful. If you give them lots of things – computers, cell phones, game stations, clothes, fancy vacations – you'll have to work such long hours to pay for it that you won't have time to spend with them. If you give them sugary cereals for breakfast, chips and cheesies at lunch, and fast food for dinner, you'll teach them your own poor dietary habits and set them on a path toward lifelong ill health.

However, health care goes beyond dietary and lifestyle choices. It also includes how you handle illness when it arises. Your great-grandparents did not give your grandparents acetaminophen every time they had a fever – they didn't have it. They also didn't have antibiotics. I'm not saying life was perfect in the good old days. Many children died of illnesses that are treatable today. We should all be grateful for the amazing advances in allopathic medicine.

But when I consider the changes in health issues and health care over the last 70 years, the most powerful message I see is that just because we can do something doesn't mean we should. Just because we can mass-produce agricultural products grown from engineered seeds planted in chemically fertilized soils doesn't mean we should. Just because we can process all the nutrients out of food to make them quick and convenient doesn't mean we should. Just because we can treat every illness with antibiotics doesn't mean we should.

As a parent, it is my belief that every time you are faced with a health care choice for your child, you should think in these terms: just because I can do this for my child, does that mean I should? Should I give my child drugs every time she's ill? Should I try to protect her from every germ? Or, should I allow symptoms of non-life-threatening illnesses to challenge her young immune systems so it can grow strong and healthy and able to cope with the challenges of occasional illness throughout her life?

What if, instead of teaching your child from the time he's a baby that sickness is bad and there's a drug for everything, you were to help him understand that there are reasons why his body spikes a fever or his sinuses get clogged with phlegm? What if you were to teach him by your example that, although the symptoms of illness are uncomfortable, they're also signs that his body is working? As a parent, you probably find it hard enough to experience symptoms of illness and put yourself to bed, instead of taking drugs and going to work so you can pay for that trip to Disneyland. It's likely even harder for you to watch your child suffer and not give them a drug to make the symptoms go away.

But when you understand how your child's body fights disease, it should become clear that giving your child drugs to alleviate every sniffle is kind of like doing his homework for him – if he doesn't do it himself, how will he learn? If you don't support his body to expel the pathogens that are making him sick, how will his body learn to do it? If you don't teach him to accept symptoms and wait the illness out, how will he ever learn how his immune system works? If you don't understand how fever works yourself, how can you teach him? Let's start there.

FEVER: THE IMMUNE SYSTEM'S FRONT LINE OF DEFENCE

No one feels good with a fever over 37–38° C (100–101° F), but a child's small body heats up quickly and there is nothing stronger than your parental instinct to protect your child. So when the doctor tells you to bring your child's fever down with a harmless drug, you do it. When the fever medication wears off, however, she feels just as bad as she did before because the germ causing her fever hasn't gone anywhere. You've made your child more comfortable, but you've also made the germs that are making her sick more comfortable.

Fever is the body's response to invasive organisms, like bacteria and viruses. These invaders don't like high temperatures. Your child's body (or yours) knows this, so when it is "invaded," her body temperature rises. At higher temperatures, viral replication slows down. This gives her immune system time to martial its forces to kick the invaders out. Those forces include cytokines (enzymes) and killer cells (white blood cells), which infiltrate the blood stream so they can seek and destroy the invaders. High body temperatures activate these cytokines and killer cells to do their jobs, so every time you bring her fever down you impede her immune system's ability to get rid of the germs that are making her sick.

Another way the immune system expels invaders is through congested sinuses or coughing. The reason your child has phlegm is that it surrounds the invading organism with a sticky glob. When he coughs, sneezes, or blows phlegm out his nose, he gets rid of the pathogens it contains. However, stuffed-up noses and hacking coughing can keep him uncomfortable and awake – and if he's awake, you're awake, too.

So you give him more over-the-counter (non-prescription or OTC) drugs, like decongestants and cough syrups. Decongestants are effective, but children can become dependent on them to continue keeping their sinuses clear. Cough syrups, on the other hand, have been proven to be literally useless. Studies have repeatedly shown a drug called dextromethorphan, commonly found in OTC cough preparations, is ineffective at recommended doses, and nobody would suggest exceeding that dosage.

I see a pattern time and time again at the clinic: a parent brings in a child with a constant runny nose or other symptoms of cold or flu. "She just seems to get over one bug, and then she gets another," says a frustrated mom. This is often because she hasn't fully recovered from the initial infection. Mom has taken the child to the doctor, looking for a prescription, but the doctor has no prescription for a virus, so he's suggested more OTC medications to suppress the child's symptoms.

But those symptoms are signs that your child's immune system is working. In generations past, your great-grandparents

95

would have monitored the fever, and perhaps brought it down with cold compresses to keep the child comfortable and prevent the fever from getting dangerously high.* When the fever broke, the virus would be gone, and the child would have developed resistance to that virus.

ANTIBIOTICS: A QUESTION OF RESISTANCE

The situation is a little different with bacterial infection. Think again about what happens when your child's body (or yours) fights infection: his temperature rises and slows down production of the invading organisms, while his body releases white blood cells and killer cells to destroy them. When you give your child medications that interfere with this process, you unintentionally create a friendlier environment for the invaders. With the immune system weakened, you go to the doctor looking for a prescription. If the illness is caused by a virus, as colds and flu are, an antibiotic will not help.

Some doctors prescribe antibiotics anyway on the theory that the viral infection may make way for a bacterial infection, and the antibiotics will prevent that. This is rarely a good idea. At times of severe illness, patients need antibiotics to help them fight infections that have gotten out of control. Antibiotics don't always destroy the infection, particularly if they're improperly used. The remaining bacteria mutate into new antibiotic-resistant strains. Improper antibiotic use has come at a cost.

Bacterial resistance to antibiotics is a serious health problem. We now have bacteria called superbugs that are resistant to some of the most powerful antibiotics ever developed. These bacteria can sometimes survive very high temperatures in the body, and can often survive longer on non-living surfaces, such as door handles and telephones, than bacteria should be able to. This is a scary situation

---

* About 1 in 25 children has at least one febrile seizure before the age of five, and about one-third have more than one. Most children outgrow them. Febrile seizures are frightening, but most are short and harmless. The main causes for concern are meningitis or a seizure disorder. The key symptom distinguishing meningitis from the flu is stiff neck. If your child has a sustained high fever and a stiff neck, go to the emergency room. If you are concerned about recurrent febrile seizures, ask your allopathic doctor to test for epilepsy or other seizure disorders. **There's no evidence that fever-lowering drugs reduce risk of seizure.** From http://www.ninds.nih.gov/disorders/febrile_seizures/detail_febrile_seizures.htm

because antibiotics can make a life-or-death difference for some patients, not only in treating contagious illnesses but in fighting infections after surgery or injury. When no other approach will defeat an infection, we need antibiotics to be effective.

When you give your child medications to reduce their symptoms, or ask a doctor to prescribe antibiotics your child doesn't need, you may feel as if you're taking control of your child's health. It's ironic that you're really contributing to a situation that takes your child's health further out of your control. It's only when you work with the illness in non-intrusive ways that your child's body will heal fully and grow strong, and you will help your child's body take control of its' health.

VACCINES AND THE PRINCIPLE OF INFORMED CONSENT

Vaccines have had an enormous impact on public health care. The efficacy of vaccinations in eradicating horrific diseases such as smallpox, polio, and tuberculosis is well documented. However, although I am happy to discuss vaccinations with patients in my clinic, I am reluctant to make blanket statements either in favour of or against vaccinations as a whole.

As with any treatment, I advise you to do your research and decide what you want for your child (or in some cases, yourself) on a case-by-case basis. Always keep in mind the principle of informed consent. You can't provide informed consent without ensuring you are fully informed.

Vaccination is an issue on which current debate is extremely heated. It is almost impossible to get a balanced perspective from any one source. This means you have to do enough research to know what questions to ask, understand the answers, and make your own decisions.

For me, the key questions about vaccines are as follows:

- *Why are there so few studies of vaccine adverse effects?* It's clear that authorities know vaccines sometimes have adverse effects from the existence of two bodies—the Vaccine Adverse Events Reporting System (VAERS) and the Vaccine Injury Compensation Program (VICP). Surely these bodies must be collecting

97

information on adverse effects. Where are the studies of these adverse effects?

- *Why are there so few studies of long-term risks?* Numerous groups such as the Vaccine Risk Awareness Network (VRAN) have collected hundreds, if not thousands, of anecdotes about healthy babies who suffered life-altering conditions after vaccination, ranging from seizure disorders and cerebral palsy to autism. How many anecdotes do we need to trigger proper studies?

- *Why do vaccine studies focus only on population health?* Much pro-vaccine information focuses on herd immunity, a theory that if 85% of a population is immunized, the unimmunized 15% will be protected. First, this is a theory, which means it's unproven; and second, it suggests that if studies could isolate individuals with risk factors for vaccine damage, those individuals could remain unimmunized without risk to others. Where are the studies of individual risk v benefit?

- *Where is the transparency in vaccine research?* Vaccine research is almost entirely funded by pharmaceutical companies with clear financial interests in promoting drugs, and public health bodies, which have their own biases toward population, rather than individual, health. Who is paying attention to these conflicts of interest in vaccine research?

- *Why do vaccine advocates fight so hard against research that looks at the issue of vaccine damage?* A few university-based researchers and independent doctors question vaccine safety. However, staunch vaccine advocates work hard at suppressing their research and even questioning their reputations. Why should researchers have to risk their careers for doing their jobs?

Please do not construe these questions as advice not to vaccinate. I do not oppose vaccination. I only question a policy of blanket vaccination undertaken without research that is specific to each individual, each vaccination, and the possible interactions between the two.

My concern regarding informed consent applies to all health issues, not only vaccination. Unfortunately, there are many situations in which patients ask questions and receive one-sided answers. This is usually true of vaccination information.[†]

Individual research is the basis of informed consent. If you do your research, you're satisfied with the answers you find, and you wish to fully comply with the recommended vaccination schedule, do what your conscience tells you to do.

On the other hand, if you want your child to be vaccinated but you have concerns about certain aspects of the vaccination schedule, you may wish to explore some of the following options:

- You could have each vaccination administered individually so you can observe reactions separately and decided on a case-by-case basis whether to continue.
- You could choose not to vaccinate against milder diseases, like chickenpox, which are certainly unpleasant, but rarely fatal.
- You could insist on using vaccines free of questionable additives, like aluminum salts and Thimerosal.[‡]
- You could consider a delayed or prolonged vaccination schedule, particularly if your infant is at risk for allergies or intolerances that have not yet emerged, or if you're simply concerned about manipulating your child's immune system before it's had time to mature.
- If your child is intolerant to eggs, you should know which vaccines are incubated in eggshells and avoid them.

There are many options. None of them are risk free. As a parent, your responsibility is to research the options and make the best choices for you and your child. That is what informed consent means. It is what personal responsibility in health is all about.

[†] In the Sources section at the back of the book, I have provided about a dozen links to information that question vaccine safety. I have, for the most part, chosen biased information to counter the pro-vaccine bias that you can find easily online without my help. To counteract this, and from an integrated medicine perspective, I have also included a link from the website of Dr. Andrew Weil, a well-respected, Harvard-educated MD and long-time practitioner of integrated medicine. He provides a pro-vaccine opinion from an integrated medicine perspective.

[‡] Aluminum salts are added to many vaccines to boost effectiveness. Several articles about this are included in the Sources. Thimerosal is a mercury-based preservative. There were so many concerns about its possible connections with autism that it is no longer used in most vaccines, but it never hurts to ask.

NUTRITION: THE BIGGEST PROBLEM IN CHILD HEALTH CARE TODAY

One of the biggest problems in child health in North America today is poor diet. The fast food industry has played a huge role in this by marketing and cross marketing directly to children, because children are pliable targets who can often influence their parents' buying decisions.

This is problematic. While many diet-related health issues are the same for children and adults, there are two important differences: first, when children establish bad habits early in life, it is much more difficult to change these habits than it is to change any habits developed in adult life. Second, children's bad habits can lay the foundation for malfunctioning body systems, so even if individuals make changes later in life, some of the harm already done will be difficult or impossible to undo.

If you have any doubt over the degree to which children's health is suffering, consider that obesity rates among Canada's children and youth have nearly tripled since the 1970s. For the first time in Canada's history, children are expected to live shorter lives than their parents because of obesity. As the following article from *Nutrition Remarks* outlines, parental attitudes factor strongly into children's behaviour:

> *It is now well known that mother's obesity status and obesogenic home environment plays a significant (possibly a synergistic) role in childhood obesity. Obese kids face both physiological and psychological challenges during childhood. Childhood obesity is known to dramatically increase the risk for heart diseases, diabetes and bone problems. Being obese is also associated with negative behavioural and physiological changes in children.*
>
> *Further, childhood obesity is a significant risk factor of child's future health in the early years and beyond. Most obese kids will be obese adults and are subsequently predisposed to type 2 diabetes, heart diseases (stroke and atherosclerosis), several types of cancer (breast, colon, endometrium, esophagus, kidney, pancreas, gall bladder,*

thyroid, ovary, cervix, and prostate cancers and multiple myeloma), and osteoarthritis.[δ]

PARENTING: MORE THAN GOOD MANNERS AND GOOD GRADES

The other important thing we role model for our children is how to manage stress. Our lives are full of it, and it has profound impacts on physical and mental health. Stress hormones impact insulin sensitivity, predisposing our bodies to obesity, diabetes, and related diseases. If stress is having an impact on our health as adults, imagine the impact it's having on our children's growing bodies.

Parenting is not only about teaching kids to have good manners, get good grades, and play well with others. Kids also need to learn about food and how to handle stress. Remember, children are like sponges: they soak up everything we show them. If we learn to take control of our own lives and health, they will learn that from us. This is what I mean by Generational Health First, which is the topic of the next chapter.

[δ] I'm sure there are reasons in this article for focusing on the mother's obesity status, but I would not wish to assign blame to mothers alone. Quote from "Relationship between Obese Moms and Kids—Epigenetics, Home Environment or Both?" *Nutrition Remarks,* May 10, 2013, http://www.nutritionremarks.com/2013/05/10/relationship-between-obese-moms-and-kids-epigenetics-home-environment-or-both/.

Chapter 10:
What Is Generational Health First?

Sometimes in the clinic, I have worked with children and adolescents, and, 10 to 15 years later, they've brought their own children to see me. Here is a very good example of what we mean by Generational Health First. In this case, I treated a teenaged girl for debilitating migraines. Her mother had taken her to their family doctor, who couldn't find a disease process underlying her symptoms and consequently prescribed drugs to relieve her symptoms.

"She's been taking hard drugs such as oxycontin and morphine," said the mother. "She's even had botox injections for pain control. This is not what I want for my teenaged daughter."

"Of course not," I said, and we began working through my algorithm. Her body composition was good, but blood tests revealed multiple food intolerances, including a significant reaction to MSG. MSG is added to many foods for flavour, but it also has an effect on insulin and blood sugar, which can trigger migraines.

"This may not be the only factor, but it's likely significant," I said to the girl. "You're going to have to alter your diet."

"Anything is better than having these migraines all the time," she said. Within a short time, she reported that her headaches had decreased by about 30%. This was good but there was room for improvement.

"Tell me more about your daily life," I said to her on a follow-up visit.

She began listing school commitments, outside activities, and social pressures. I'm amazed by the amount of stress in many teenagers' lives. Her stress levels were extraordinarily high and it showed in urinary cortisol levels that were fine during the day, but high at night.

"Is that why I have a hard time falling asleep?" She asked.

"It could be," I said. "Cortisol should spike in the morning to give you the boost you need to start the day, level off over the afternoon to keep you going through the day, and drop in the evening to allow you to unwind. If you're not sleeping well because of high cortisol, lack of sleep could be contributing to your headaches."

An intravenous combination of vitamins, minerals, and botanicals stabilized her cortisol levels and reduced the frequency of her headaches by another 25%. I then recommended some physical therapies, such as massage, physiotherapy, and posture awareness to help reduce her physical tension.

In another conversation, I asked for more specific details about her eating habits, exercise routines, and menstrual cycle. This led to analyses of her blood sugar and reproductive hormones. I ruled out premenstrual tension, but then I questioned her further about meals.

"I get busy and forget to eat sometimes," she admitted.

By the time I finished with this patient, although the severity of her headaches hadn't changed much, the frequency had been reduced by 60% or more. These were life-altering results for her, allowing her to have fun at a time in life that everyone should be able to enjoy.

What was even more interesting to me was the Generational Health First aspect of this story. Ten years later, this teenager was a young woman who had married and had a daughter of her own. When the child was still quite young, the new mom brought her in to be tested for food intolerances. After expressing delight at how well she was doing, I asked whether her daughter had any particular symptoms.

"No," she said, "but I don't want to wait for symptoms to develop. I want to know if she has any problems I should watch for. I went through years of headaches and painkillers before you helped me."

"I don't blame my mom," she said. "She didn't know. But I do. And I'll do anything to protect my little girl from what I went through."

PREVENTION, NOT PALLIATION

When I talk about Generational Health First, I am referring the idea of making a preventive approach to health part of the family knowledge and heritage that gets passed down to the next generation. At present, this is something most of us have to think about deliberately, but my goal is for it to become such an integral aspect of life that our grandchildren will pass it along to their children and grandchildren without even thinking about it.

That sounds great! How do we get there from here?

The same way we got so many people to quit smoking, which was good, and to eat a low-fat diet, which was not so good – one person at a time. And it starts with you. Now that you have some educational background, the rest of this book will focus on a sort of roadmap you can follow to begin making generational health your first priority. It starts with each of us taking control of our own health.

What exactly is the naturopathic definition of health?

In naturopathic medicine, we see optimal health as a balance between the biological, psychological, and social factors in our lives. They all play significant, interlocking roles in human health and disease.

Is this what you mean by the mind-body connection?

Yes. Dr. Candace Pert, an internationally recognized pharmacologist who has published over 250 scientific articles, wrote early in her career (in the 1980s) that "most psychologists treat the mind as disembodied, a phenomenon with little or no connection to the physical body. Conversely, most physicians treat the body with no regard to the mind or the emotions. But the body and mind are not separate, and we cannot treat one without the other."* Pert's main areas of research connected neuropeptides, which are short chains of amino acids in the brain, with emotions, on one hand, and the immune system, on the other hand.

---

* This quote was taken directly from Dr. Candace Pert's website at http://candacepert.com/. Pert died unexpectedly in 2012. Her website has since been suspended.

How did the roles of the body and mind in health become disconnected?

That goes back even earlier than the Industrial Revolution to a 17th-century philosopher named René Descartes. There was some dispute in medieval Europe between early scientists and the Roman Catholic Church about what scientists should be allowed to question, and what should be left to God. Descartes resolved the issue by claiming that the body was physical and therefore could be studied scientifically without going against God's will, but the mind was metaphysical and therefore belonged to religion.

From there, western science and medicine evolved to study the body, in isolation from the mind. Pert tried to heal this divide by showing that our emotions are based in chemical reactions in our brains, and can trigger physical processes that affect our health.

Do allopathic doctors acknowledge the mind-body connection?

Allopathic doctors have begun to recognize that the body and mind work together, but allopathic treatments are still rooted in differential diagnosis. As a result, many allopathic diagnoses, and the pharmaceutical treatments prescribed for them, focus on the body as if it operates separately from the mind. This is why I believe it's important to understand the history of modern medicine, the 3 Ps, and the difference between prevention and palliation. These are all ways of understanding the concept of Generational Health First.

As naturopathic doctors, we look at the whole person, including their disease history, to assess their risk of chronic degenerative diseases like cancer and arthritis. Rather than wait for symptoms to appear, we carry out tests to help us predict the likelihood that they will occur. We perform tests to confirm the presence of disease, such as diabetes, when appropriate, as an allopathic doctor would, but we prefer to see patients before diseases have developed and help them transform bad health habits into good ones to avoid developing the disease.

Unfortunately, that's not always possible. There are times when people do all the right things, but genetic factors are so powerful they develop diabetes or have a heart attack anyway. But by caring for their health well, they may delay the development of a disease, or minimize its severity.

So allopathic doctors wait to see if patients get sick instead of offering preventive treatment?

There's more to it than that. Sometimes people have symptoms they can describe, but there isn't a diagnosis to go along with their symptoms. In allopathic medicine, it's difficult to treat symptoms without a diagnosis. At that point, some doctors will simply say there's nothing wrong and send the patient on their way. This can be frustrating to a patient who knows something is wrong. Other doctors will believe the patient, but without a diagnosis, they have few options but to follow a palliative protocol, which may have either immediate or long-term adverse effects. Many doctors will believe the patient, but still find some way to explain away the symptoms without looking for an underlying cause.

Like when the doctor told the retired businessman his symptoms were inevitable signs of aging?

Yes. They were signs of aging, but they weren't inevitable. Still other times, a doctor will diagnose a patient's symptoms as signs of depression and treat her with antidepressants instead of seeking an underlying problem. Or the doctor may say a patient is malingering, which means making up symptoms because they want something in return, like attention or financial compensation.

NO MORE US-AND-THEM

I don't want to give the impression of an us-and-them attitude between naturopathic and allopathic doctors. As I described earlier, there was a lot of that in my student years. After over nearly 30 years of practice, I've realized there is a place and a need for different kinds of health care, and I've seen positive signs that many allopathic doctors are recognizing this, too. In fact, there is significant overlap in what naturopathic and allopathic doctors do. Look at the chart called "Naturopathic and Allopathic Care: A Comparison." This clearly shows differences and similarities in the ways allopathic and naturopathic doctors approach health, but I hope it also shows that both disciplines have equally vital roles to play in our health care system.

106

To provide a final illustration of generational health first, I'm going to close this section with another story. Then I encourage you to go on to Part II and read about Dr. Jheeta's Algorithm, a systematic approach to naturopathic health care. It's a step-by-step protocol I use to evaluate each new patient's current state of health, uncover issues underlying the symptoms that brought them to me, predict their risk of developing chronic degenerative disease in the future, and recommend steps they might take to eliminate existing symptoms and reduce risk.

This is not a revolutionary idea. It's an approach all properly educated naturopathic doctors use in one way or another, although they don't all call it Dr. Jheeta's Algorithm. My goal in writing it down for everyone to see and use is to help people understand that naturopathic doctors are fully trained, primary care physicians who bring a different perspective to health care than allopathic doctors, – a perspective that focuses on prevention rather than palliation. As I realized in my fourth year of naturopathic college, these approaches work best when they work together. I may have begun college with an us-and-them attitude to allopathic medicine, but I've long since realized it has no place anywhere in health care.

NATUROPATHIC AND ALLOPATHIC CARE: A COMPARISON

Naturopathic Care	Allopathic Care
Health is a balance between the mind and the body.	Health is the absence of symptoms of disease.
Being unhealthy is an imbalance or disharmony of natural body energy.	Being unhealthy results from a defect of the bodily structure with a cause and symptoms.
Symptoms are the body's way of showing that it wants to heal and needs help.	Symptoms are a sign of illness and must be eliminated or suppressed.
The cause of an illness is any action that will cause an imbalance in the mind, body, or spirit.	An abnormal condition of a part, organ, or system of an organism resulting from various causes, such as infection, inflammation, environmental factors or genetic.

The patient's responsibility is to prevent illness and live a healthy lifestyle.	The patient's responsibility is to see the doctor when something needs healing.
Tests are performed to assess wellness as well as sickness.	Tests are performed to determine whether illness is present, or assess level of illness.
The doctor's role is to assist people in staying well.	The doctor's role is to assist people when they are ill or injured.
The goal of treatment is to restore balance through lifestyle changes and other natural means.	The goal of treatment is to suppress symptoms, usually through drugs or surgery.
The main strength is the focus on prevention and management of chronic illness and the recognition of the importance of lifestyle and the mind-body connection.	The main strength is the ability to treat structural trauma and defects and address life-threatening illnesses that require medical or surgical intervention.

GENERATIONAL HEALTH FIRST: OUR MISSION STATEMENT IN A STORY

In the first few years of my practice, one of my patients was a mother who'd been coping with numerous health concerns since her daughter's birth eight years earlier. She had not lost all her pregnancy weight, she was struggling with IBS, she was tired all the time, and she had become depressed from the stress of her health issues.

Her daughter was having health issues as well. She'd been a colicky baby, which means she'd had digestive issues from the start. She had extensive eczema, struggled with a moderate sleep disorder, and was constantly tired and irritable.

"I've been to several doctors for myself," the mother told me. "And I've taken my daughter to several doctors. I'm not getting any answers. I've tried to lose the weight. I'm not sure why nothing is working. I've applied one skin cream after another to my daughter's skin and her eczema never clears up. I've been told to train her to sleep through the night by letting her cry it out alone, but her tummy is hurting and her skin is itchy and sore, so I'm not surprised she can't sleep. Isn't there a better way?"

I started by taking her history, and found out, not surprisingly, that the mother had learned her dietary habits from her parents, who'd tell her to fill her plate with food and finish her dinner even if she was full. They fed her a standard Canadian diet rich in refined sugar, white flour, processed fat, and refined salt. Her whole family was obese.

I began working through the algorithm with her by offering suggestions for better food choices and portion sizes. Then I tested her for food intolerances to see if they could be contributing to her IBS. Over the next few months, she eliminated the offending foods from her diet and followed a strict course of supplements I prescribed to improve her gut health.

On her next visit, she said, "I must have lost weight because my clothes are feeling looser. I'm not feeling so bloated and gassy. I have more energy to get up in the morning."

Naturally, she was eager to have this protocol applied to her young daughter. In very little time, we began to see improvements in her skin and lessening of her digestive issues. The mother was happier, the daughter was healthier, and we left things at that.

Over 20 years later, a new patient walked into my office but looked awfully familiar. It was the eight-year-old daughter who was now 29 with a baby boy of her own.

"It's so nice to see you," I said. "You look wonderful."

"Thank you," she said. "I've always remembered what a difference you made to our lives. My mom lost more weight and kept it off, and I've never had another problem with eczema or any other health problem, other than the occasional cold or flu. But my little boy is a bit colicky, so I wanted you to screen him for food intolerances and find out if there's anything I should be taking out of his diet or any supplements you think he might need."

"It will be my pleasure," I said. "You are exactly what we mean when we talk about making generational health our first priority. You're the best advertising my clinic could have. You're the best advertising my whole profession could have!"

This young woman's mother had taken all my advice to heart, and lived it from that point on. It had changed the course of her life, and her daughter's life.

It took me nearly 30 years to develop the approach I was building early in my practice, an approach that really had its start during my fourth year in naturopathic college. That approach is the system I now call Dr. Jheeta's Algorithm.

It doesn't need to take you 30 years to understand Dr. Jheeta's Algorithm. Now that I've provided what I think are the key bits of information you need to understand how it works, all you have to do to begin putting it to work for yourself is turn the page.

PART II: EVALUATION

INTRODUCTION

Becoming more accountable for our own and our family's health can seem like a huge task, but it doesn't have to be. We all learned to walk by taking small steps, and we can learn to take back control of our health in the same way. One way to start is with a simple mental exercise.

Sit in a comfortable spot, close your eyes, and think about the last time you felt truly healthy. How old were you? Were you a teenager, or in your twenties? Were you eating three meals per day without any digestive problems? Were you sleeping well and waking up energized each morning, happy and ready for a new day? Did you have fewer worries about things like relationships and money? Try to remember how great you felt and reconnect with the feeling of being truly healthy.

When and how did you stop feeling this way? If you're like many people, the shift happened gradually. As money and family matters became higher priorities, you began taking your health for granted. You didn't realize that when you sacrifice your health – even if it is to earn money and do other important things for yourself and your family – fatigue and stress can creep in and become part of your daily life. Small symptoms can begin to appear. You may notice you've been tired, or have had indigestion, but you keep thinking, "It's no big deal. I can handle it." So, you buy another bottle of antacid and learn to live with it.

If this sounds like you, then by this point in the book, you might be getting the idea that these recurring symptoms, no matter how small you think they are, can signal the beginning of chronic health problems. This knowledge gives you a choice: to go on as you are and wait until your symptoms turn into chronic illness, and then take palliative measures to manage your symptoms, or to take a few steps now to prevent your symptoms from turning into chronic disease.

As you learn about your health and our health care system, I hope you will decide to take responsibility for your health by opting for prevention before palliation whenever possible. I hope you will choose to trade in bad health habits for good ones. And I hope you will do it not only for yourself, but also for the next generation of children, and every one after that.

To make this choice as easy as possible, I've created a simple tool to help you understand what's going on with your health today and take some control over how you'd like your health to be in the future. I call this tool: Dr. Jheeta's Algorithm.

Dr. Jheeta's Algorithm is a simple system you can use to assess what's happening with your health now, discuss changes you might make with your health care provider, and have confidence that your choices will deliver results.

Dr. Jheeta's Algorithm includes five levels of evaluation that help me estimate a patient's risk for some of the top chronic diseases in the world today. You may not be able to use it in exactly the same way, but you certainly can use it as a guide to help you recognize the warning signs of conditions like heart disease, diabetes, arthritis, various cancers, depression, and many others, and use that awareness to take control of your health before disease strikes.

Disclaimer: I am NOT suggesting you abandon the advice of your MD or any other health care provider. The evaluations and testing methods I describe in Part II, and any other part of the book are in no way designed to replace the advice or practices of your allopathic physician or other health care professional. I wrote this book for the educational purposes of a mass audience. There is no way for myself or this book to individually diagnose or treat a patient's condition without an in-person evaluation at my clinic.

CHAPTER 11:
DR. JHEETA'S ALGORITHM

Have you ever had your cortisol levels tested? Do you know why it's important to test insulin levels as well as blood sugar levels? Have you had toxic load testing, or been evaluated for food intolerances? Do you know the difference between your biological age and your chronological age?

In my practice, I've found very few people have had these simple tests. Yet, the results of tests like these can provide critical information about your current health status. They can provide a baseline that represents where you are now, and what adjustments you might make to your diet, exercise routine, or stress management practices to minimize your risk of developing a chronic health issue.

For example, did you know that as we age many biological markers also change, biological markers like nutrients and hormones just to name a few? By monitoring these values we can try and predict if a patient is aging at an accelerated rate. We can teach our patients how to manage these markers and stabilize the aging process hopefully to improve their health, well-being and longevity without necessarily treating any specific disease at all.

This type of evaluation method can help you understand how healthy you are today, as opposed to how sick you are, so we can really focus on true prevention instead of early detection of disease. I can't emphasize enough the difference here: early detection allows for a greater chance of recovery, however, the disease process has now been well established. I believe true prevention can address disease well before it is established.

Now please refer to the chart – Figure #1 on page 115. Don't worry about understanding it now. As I explain the algorithm, you can follow along with this chart to better understand how it works. I have developed my

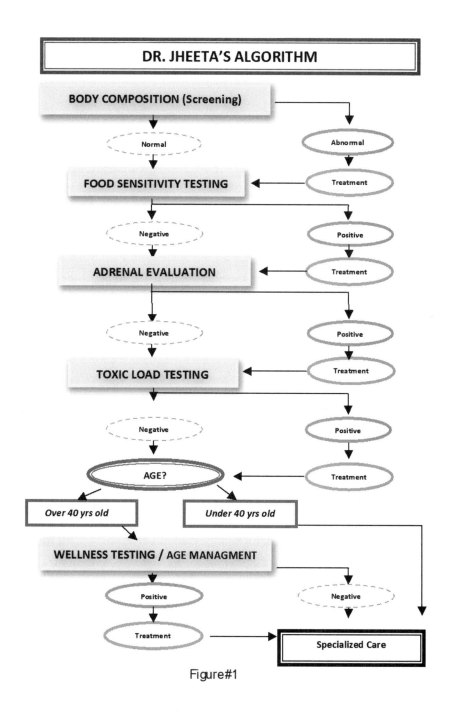

Figure#1

algorithm over nearly three decades of observing and treating thousands of patients at my clinic. I use it every day because it represents the most logical order for evaluating and treating people who come to my clinic with their health concerns.

The algorithm helps me predict how likely it is that a patient will become ill without treatment. I base my predictions on my daily practical experience and the results I have achieved by using this system over and over again. The order of the evaluations and recommended treatments in the algorithm is very important. It starts with body composition, the foundation of health, and builds through five levels of assessment, culminating with an evaluation of how the patient's body is handling the aging process. Many of the worst diseases that plague us today are considered inevitable aspects of aging, but I believe many of them are preventable, if patients take the right steps.

FIVE LEVELS OF EVALUATION

First, I do a Body Composition Evaluation. Most chronic diseases are directly connected to diet, exercise, and body measurements, which research has proven to be more important than weight. As I've discussed, refined sugar, processed fats, and refined salt are three of the biggest contributors to problems with body composition. Exercise is also a significant factor, which I will discuss in Chapter 20.

Second, I perform a Food Intolerance Evaluation. I've had many patients whose lives have been transformed simply by becoming aware of their food intolerances. I test for food intolerances with blood tests and functional testing, which allows patients to learn how their foods may be interacting with their bodies, possibly leading to immune system dysfunction and even initiating disease processes.

Third, I do an Adrenal Evaluation. An Adrenal Evaluation can also be described as a stress evaluation since each of us is under some kind of stress virtually all the time. Stress in moderation can be good for health, but the constant presence of stress hormones can trigger serious health problems. In the clinic, I assess a patient's stress levels by measuring levels of a hormone called cortisol, and by checking the function of the adrenal gland by measuring other adrenal hormones. Checking these levels at various times of the day can help me determine whether a patient's symptoms might be stress related.

Fourth, I perform a Toxic Load Evaluation. Allopathic medicine recognizes and treats acute exposure to toxins, but in naturopathic medicine, we have found that long-term low-level exposure can cause toxic metals to build up in body tissues over time. Some patients have no reaction to this build-up, while others have symptoms ranging from fatigue or headaches to chronic inflammation. If I know about toxicity, I can offer treatment to eliminate toxins from the body.

Fifth, I perform a Wellness Evaluation, also known as Age Management Testing. There is no such thing as reversing the aging process. However, numerous naturally occurring proteins and hormones in our bodies can serve as markers of aging processes. If testing detects any of these markers are at lower than I'd expect to see in a person of the patient's chronological age, I can offer supplements to elevate them and bring a person's biological age back in line with his or her chronological age.

I perform these tests in this order for specific reasons. I check body composition first because it is the single most common factor in patients' chronic health issues. I check food intolerances second because we cannot escape our need for food, but are often unaware that particular foods may cause specific reactions. Some patients, and other NDs, question why I check stress third, as stress is often an underlying factor in food intolerances. It can seem arbitrary, but I feel it's important to identify food intolerances before considering whether they are the problem, or simply a symptom of stress.

I leave toxic load closer to the end of the algorithm because symptoms of chronic exposure tend to be rare. It makes sense to rule out more common causes before continuing to something that's less likely. I test for age management last because often, if age is a factor, a disease process has already manifested and the patient is under the care of an allopathic doctor. It's uncommon for a patient to arrive at my clinic in generally good health but with a few complaints related to premature aging, thought it does happen occasionally.

YOU DON'T HAVE TO BE SICK TO BENEFIT

I usually work through the algorithm with patients who come to me with specific symptoms. However, I encourage you to use the algorithm, or as much of it as you can, with the help of a qualified naturopath, to evaluate your own health today, even if you are feeling good. This will enable you to work proactively to incorporate preventive thinking into your daily routine. As you read through the algorithm, you may realize you've been ignoring minor symptoms, which may be your body's way of saying you have left a problem too long. Paying attention to these messages in the present may help you prevent chronic health issues from arising in the future.

CHAPTER 12:
BODY COMPOSITION EVALUATION

Dr. Jheeta's Algorithm begins with a Body Composition Evaluation. When addressing body composition, I look for a combination of physical appearance, attitude toward diet, food portioning (how much you eat at a meal), and exercise. This evaluation can be a powerful way to identify your risk of conditions such as heart disease, diabetes, arthritis, and some cancers.

You may have heard of a method of measuring body composition called Body Mass Index (BMI). BMI has been the standard method used for many years, but it fails to consider that excessive body weight is not always fat. If you are short and stocky, the BMI might say you are overweight, when in fact you eat well, work out regularly, and your body is solid muscle.

I use the BMI at times, but I don't rely on it to evaluate body composition. Instead, I use a simple combination of body measurements: chest-to-waist measurements for men, and waist-to-hip measurements for women. Ideally, a man's chest should be larger than his waist, and a woman's hips should be larger than her waist.

BELLY FAT

To get even more specific we are talking about belly fat. Belly fat doesn't just lay idle at your beltline. Researchers describe this large mass as an active "organ" in your body – one that churns out hormones and inflammatory substances.

High belly fat is associated with known diseases such as hypertension, diabetes, and high cholesterol (hypercholesterolemias). It is also associated with increased arterial disease including atherosclerosis and arteriosclerosis. In one study, men with excess belly fat and a large waist were most at risk for what researchers call "all-cause mortality" – early death from any cause. Belly fat metabolism causes fatty acid to drain into the liver, which can cause a whole host of diseases from blood clots to strokes to insulin resistance leading to diabetes and even links to certain cancers.

We need to be careful here not to overreact to the idea that excess belly fat and other fat, or what many would call excess body weight, should be used as the sole means of assessing one's health, as this idea seems to result in instances where people feel they need to consider extreme dieting! The idea that an extreme diet can result in weight loss due to muscle and fat loss where a person may appear to look healthy based on this extreme diet regime, is however, in many cases false. As this person might also have a poor muscle to fat ratio and still have a high level of visceral fat (intra abdominal fat), which is associated with most of the unhealthy consequences of obesity!

Having excess fat on the inside and a normal appearance on the outside can increase the risk of disease similar to those who look overtly overweight. This is very important when you consider that a good assessment of obesity is a measurement of waist circumference. So it's clear that reducing central obesity is important; however, how you decrease this obesity is just as important. Extreme dieting and borderline starvation is definitely not the answer. A well planned protocol to reduce central obesity efficiently while spurring muscle mass is ideal. Consequently, these protocols require careful thought and planning, which is where we use our referral network to help direct certain cases to appropriate, endorsed weight management professionals: something we get into in the Empowerment section of this book.

THE RIGHT MEASUREMENTS MEAN THE BEST RESULTS

You may look in the mirror and say, "hey, I look great!" But it's better to rely on a tape measure, as the numbers don't lie. Try not to focus on exact measurements, but proportion. If you're a man, your chest should be at least an inch larger than your waist. And if you're a woman, your hips should be at least an inch larger than your waist.

When I begin a body composition evaluation, some patients tell me they have a slow metabolism. This is true in some cases. It could be caused by prescription medications, stress, or hereditary factors. If you are concerned about this, I suggest you make an appointment with a naturopathic doctor to identify and treat any metabolic reasons for poor body composition, such as thyroid problems.

But, for 90% of my patients this just isn't the case. In most cases, reducing food intake and increasing exercise levels will increase daily metabolic rate, where your body is burning and using calories efficiently. The best way to reduce calories is by cutting out refined sugars and fats, and developing a regular exercise routine, but I'll discus that more in Chapter 20.

Experience has shown the importance of taking body composition measurements right before proceeding with other evaluations. If you take body measurements incorrectly, the traditional tests for blood pressure, blood sugar, and cholesterol, may be of little use.

Chapter 13:
Food Intolerance Evaluation

The next step in Dr. Jheeta's Algorithm is a Food Intolerance Evaluation. If you have completed a Body Composition Evaluation and you are still experiencing symptoms, they may be caused by a food intolerance. The following symptoms may suggest food intolerances:

- Digestive pains and discomfort, such as cramps, bloating, diarrhea, constipation, or nausea,
- Musculoskeletal problems, such as pain, stiffness, and swelling,
- Skin problems, such as dryness, rashes, redness, swelling, and itching,
- Nervous system problems, such as fatigue or headaches,
- Respiratory problems, such as shallow breathing or shortness of breath,
- Endocrine system (hormone regulation) problems, such as inexplicable weight gain or loss.

Three common issues we see at the clinic that are often related to food intolerances are migraine headaches, eczema, and irritable bowel syndrome (IBS). If you have eczema, you may have been taking drugs ranging from antihistamines to corticosteroids, and applying topical corticosteroid creams. While these can help relieve symptoms, they do not address underlying causes.

If you have chronic migraines, you have been managing them for as long as possible with aspirin, acetaminophen, and ibuprofen. However, when these over-the-counter (OTC) analgesics become ineffective, you may have little choice but to proceed to addictive drugs, such as oxycontin or morphine, or you may already have taken that step.

If you have been diagnosed with irritable bowel syndrome (IBS), you have my sympathy. IBS is not the name of a disease but a description of bowel behaviour. You may have been prescribed drugs to slow your bowels down during attacks of diarrhea, or to speed them up during episodes of constipation; you may take anti-flatulents to reduce gas, or steroids to reduce inflammation; and you may have been told you need surgical intervention, or you may already have taken that step.

Although eczema, migraines, and IBS seem like very different health issues, patients who have them experience one common symptom: severe, recurring bouts of frustration because drugs only help them manage their symptoms without getting at underlying causes or lasting cures. These three problems, in particular, are often caused by food intolerances.

"SOMETIMES IT BOTHERS ME, OTHER TIMES IT DOESN'T"

In the clinic, I evaluate food intolerances initially with a blood test. This helps me determine how your immune system reacts to certain foods; reactions could be anywhere from mild to severe. In most cases, I can determine what you should and should not eat, and often which foods you can and cannot safely combine.

Many patients say to me, "sometimes, when I eat this food, it bothers me, but other times it doesn't." If you have ever noticed this, you may be eating two foods to which you are intolerant at the same time, not realizing you are sensitive to both. Your body may be able to cope with mild intolerances one at a time, but triggering multiple reactions at the same time can layer on too much stress and cause symptoms.

Many people live most of their lives with food intolerances. Because they don't have immediate, overt symptoms, such as anaphylaxis, or because their reactions don't show up for 24, 48, or even 72 hours after they've eaten the food, they don't make the connection. If you have just assumed that any unpleasant symptoms you've been having are the way things are for everyone, a food intolerance evaluation may help.

DRAMATIC CHANGE FOR THE BETTER

The blood test I perform provides a starting place. Based on the results, I will provide a list of foods for you to completely eliminate until all your symptoms resolve. You will then begin reintroducing foods one at a time for three days, up to three times a day.

If a problem occurs, you will remove that food from your diet, wait for symptoms to resolve, and try the next one. If there is no exacerbation of symptoms, you will move forward to check another intolerance for three days. Any time problems re-occur, you will eliminate the most recently added food. Occasionally, you may need to introduce a food twice to make sure you are not getting false positives.

Once problem foods have been identified, I will suggest you avoid foods to which you are highly intolerant, and avoid combining foods to which you are mildly to moderately intolerant. If you have multiple intolerances, where total avoidance may not be practical, I may suggest you try a rotation diet. I describe this in more detail in Chapter 21.

The changes patients experience as a result of the Food Intolerance Evaluation are often dramatic. Patients whose diarrhea sometimes forced them to stay close to a toilet are able to leave the house again. Patients who have been wearing concealing clothing to cover up skin rashes may enjoy wearing shorts and baring their arms in warm weather.

Patients who have undergone this type of evaluation and enjoyed relief from years of symptoms do not forget their experience. They often recommend the same procedure, advice, education, or treatment to friends and family members. Many patients who benefit from a food intolerance evaluation when they are children or teens come back years later with their own child. The child may not have symptoms yet, but the parent may wish to do some preventive work.

This is Generational Health First at its best.

CHAPTER 14:
ADRENAL EVALUATION (STRESS)

The next step in Dr. Jheeta's Algorithm is the Adrenal Evaluation, more commonly known as a Stress Evaluation. Many patients come to the clinic with a long list of ambiguous symptoms, which can be very difficult to diagnose. This list could go on for pages, and I offer a somewhat more detailed list in Chapter 22, but the stress symptoms I see most often at the clinic include:

- Fatigue,
- Insomnia,
- Headaches or migraines,
- Digestive issues, including nausea, diarrhea, constipation, abnormal stools, or cramping,
- Skin problems, including rashes, eczema, lesions, or acne,
- Hair conditions, including excessive hair growth or hair loss,
- Mental wellness issues, such as depression or anxiety,
- Specific food intolerances.

Many of the above symptoms are the same ones we test for with a Food Intolerance Evaluation. This is what I mean by "ambiguous": these symptoms could be caused by any number of problems. The only way to determine the cause is through evaluation consisting of a process of elimination and identification. After body composition and food intolerances, the next step is an Adrenal Evaluation.

IT IS ALL IN YOUR HEAD, SO LET'S FOCUS ON THAT

If you have a long list of symptoms like these, you may be frustrated because your allopathic doctors have said, "I can't find anything wrong with you" and prescribed antidepressants or referred you to a psychiatrist. Either way, from a psychiatric perspective, your symptoms are likely to be considered signs of depression and, although treatment may include counselling, it is also likely to include drugs.

Depression is a serious illness and many patients benefit from antidepressant drugs. However, antidepressants are sometimes prescribed when a patient has persistent symptoms of stress. Stress is not a specific illness that an allopathic doctor can define with differential diagnosis, but as I've seen many times in my practice, there isn't always an illness to diagnose. Out-of-control stress can often cause anxiety and depression. Whether the outcome of your stress is chronic fatigue, migraines, IBS, or depression, anti-depressant drugs may seem to help, but they can often mask symptoms, making it impossible to get at the root of them.

Television ads for anti-depressants typically depict a woman who can't get out of bed to spend time with her young child, or a man who has stopped enjoying his work and being productive. They take the medication and fling open the curtains to let the sun in, play with their children, contribute enthusiastically to meetings, and joke around at work, but antidepressants don't automatically make people happy, as the commercials suggest. Moreover, they can cause adverse effects, in both the short and long term. In addition, if underlying stress causes the depression, the same stress can contribute to other chronic conditions over the long term.

CORTISOL AND ADRENAL TESTING: REAL LIFE SAVERS

I begin the Adrenal Evaluation with a questionnaire, which serves as a starting point for discussion. I would then begin cortisol testing and send you home with instructions to take saliva samples at four defined intervals over an 18-hour period, along with urine samples at four defined intervals over a 24-hour period. The salivary test is an excellent, non-invasive way to measure cortisol, and therefore assess stress levels. The urine test complements this by providing a more complete picture of adrenal function.

If you are healthy, your cortisol levels should have a distinct cycle. They should be lower at night, allowing you to sleep comfortably. They should spike in the early morning, which helps you wake up energized for the new day. Through the afternoon, they should level out, allowing you to maintain focus. Then they should drop in the evening, so you can prepare for sleep again.

Cortisol levels provide a measurable way of showing that the connection between mind and body is not imaginary, but very real. Accurate evaluation is the key to empowerment, and empowerment is the key to making changes, letting go of bad habits, and creating good ones to replace them. A crucial part of this is recognizing stressors and understanding how they are affecting your overall health.

If you are experiencing abnormal levels of cortisol and other markers of adrenal function, I will initiate a number of naturopathic protocols to restore your body to a healthy state. However, a vital part of restoring health will be recognizing and managing the causes of your stress, which I will discuss more fully in Chapter 22.

After six to eight weeks, I will do a second series of saliva and urine tests to determine if your cortisol levels and overall adrenal function have returned to more stable, normal levels. If they have, but you are still experiencing symptoms, we may move on to testing for toxic load.

CHAPTER 15:
TOXIC LOAD EVALUATION

The next step in Dr. Jheeta's Algorithm is Toxic Load Evaluation. Over the course of your life, you have more than likely been exposed to many harmful toxins, both organic and inorganic. These toxins can accumulate in your body over time, contributing to toxic load, a build-up of molecules that are foreign and harmful to your body. Toxic load may be related to a wide array of health problems, including:

- Cardiovascular diseases (heart attack)
- Cerebrovascular diseases (stroke)
- Neurodegenerative diseases (such as Parkinson's and Alzheimer's diseases)
- Immunologic diseases (such as arthritis, thyroiditis, chronic infections)

Low-level toxic load is not well recognized in allopathic medicine. However, in naturopathic medicine we have a different approach. We use standard laboratory tests to evaluate toxic load, and remove toxins without harming your body.

THE DETOXIFICATION PROCESS

In the clinic, I would begin the Toxic Load Evaluation by asking questions to obtain a better understanding of what symptoms you are experiencing. If we have already worked through the first three levels of the Algorithm, I will decide on the basis of the information gained from those levels and any additional information you are providing at this stage whether to draw blood and assess your toxic load.

Depending on the degree of toxicity and a few other factors, I will follow one of two principle paths: direct or indirect detoxification therapy. Direct treatment involves removing toxins using chelation therapy, while indirect treatment helps the body detoxify itself by supporting liver function. The following is a succinct definition of chelation therapy available on the website of Dr. Andrew Weil[*]:

> *Chelation therapy is a treatment used in conventional medicine for removing heavy metals (including mercury) from the blood. It involves intravenous injections of a chelating agent, EDTA, a synthetic amino acid. EDTA binds to heavy metals and minerals in the blood so that they can be excreted in the urine. Another intravenous agent used by some physicians for mercury detoxification is called DMPS.*
>
> *An oral chelating agent called Succimer is FDA-approved for treatment of lead poisoning and is used by some physicians to remove mercury from the body. The drug combines with metals in the bloodstream and then both the metals and the drug are removed from the body by the kidneys and then excreted. Common side effects include diarrhea, loose stools, nausea and vomiting, poor appetite and skin rash.* [†]

Indirect detoxification protocols are less invasive. If your toxic load seems less severe, I may choose indirect detoxification, which involves oral administration of some of the same agents used in chelation therapy or minerals such as selenium and glutathione, which facilitate the same process. Like chelation therapy, the intent is for the toxins in your body to bind to the molecules of the detoxification agent and to be flushed out of your system in your urine. Indirect detoxification takes place in two phases. In phase I, the liver processes a toxin into a non-toxic product, while in phase II it converts it into a water-soluble form to be excreted through the urine.

I often recommend my patients supplement detoxification techniques with supportive therapies such as infrared sauna and hydrotherapy. Infrared sauna is a type of sauna that provokes sweat,

---

[*] Andrew Weil, MD, is a widely respected physician who combines a Harvard education with 40 years of practising *integrated medicine*. Integrated medicine is a way of combining the best of a wide variety of approaches to health care, including allopathic and naturopathic medicine, and other health care modalities.

[†] "Chelation Therapy," Dr. Andrew Weil, *Weil,*
http://www.drweil.com/drw/u/ART03408/Chelation-Therapy.html.

through which more toxins may be eliminated, without the high heat of other types of saunas. The principle behind using hydrotherapy (a hot tub) is the same. Both infrared saunas and hot tubs are available in many community-based locations.

In most cases I continue the recommended protocols with the goal of maintaining low toxic load for six to eight weeks, and then reassess the chief complaint. If I see acceptable improvements, I will likely suggest you continue treatment for six months, and then I will take another blood test to reassess toxic load and determine whether there is anything further you need from me.

CHAPTER 16:
WELLNESS OR AGE MANAGEMENT EVALUATION

Wellness Evaluation is the fifth and final stage of Dr. Jheeta's Algorithm. I also refer to this as Age Management Testing. As described in Chapter 8, certain markers of health, such as various growth hormones, sex hormones, proteins, and enzymes, change as we age. These changes can cause a variety of symptoms, such as:

- Overall decrease in energy and vigor,
- Tendency to become easily tired,
- Changes in sleeping patterns,
- Deteriorating memory,
- Unexplained behavioral changes,
- Skin changes, such as wrinkles, brown spots, or loss of skin elasticity on the limbs,
- Hair loss or changes in hair color,
- Deteriorating vision or hearing,
- Changes in bowel function,
- Decreased libido,
- Sexual dysfunction,
- Urinary problems such as incontinence, dribbling, or changes in frequency of urination,
- Changes in menstrual cycle,
- Abdominal obesity and inability to lose weight.

DON'T ACT THE AGE YOU FEEL; FEEL THE AGE YOU ARE!

Many people, including most allopathic doctors, treat these symptoms as inevitable aspects of aging. In naturopathic medicine, we don't agree they have to be. We all have certain aches and pains as time goes on, but if you are experiencing troubling symptoms that seem out of place for your chronological age, there is often something I can do to address them.

Even more importantly, these symptoms can indicate that a chronic degenerative disease is in the early stages of development. Measuring these markers of age can help me predict the likelihood that a chronic disease will manifest, act to prevent it, delay its onset, reverse its early effects, or at least slow its progression.

To do this, I use the Wellness or Age Management Evaluation. This involves taking a blood test and sending it to a laboratory to have levels of the hormones and proteins identified in Chapter 8 analyzed. When the results come back, I will compare them with standard measures for your chronological age. If your levels indicate premature signs of aging, I may prescribe a variety of nutraceutical supplements to correct them.

However, this level of testing is really only useful for people over 40 years of age. If you are under 40 and I have been unable to address your health concerns through the first four evaluations, there is little chance I will find relevant information through a Wellness or Age Management Evaluation. You are simply not old enough to be experiencing the hormonal or other fluctuations that occur with age. In this case, I will continue evaluating and treating you under a different category, which I'll discuss in Chapter 18.

CHAPTER 17:
DR. JHEETA'S ALGORITHM FOR CHILDREN

Because I feel so strongly about the importance of a generational attitude toward health care, I have created a slightly modified form of the algorithm for children. Dr. Jheeta's Algorithm for children is much like the algorithm for adults, but with three steps instead of five: body composition, food intolerances, and toxic load.

I don't do a stress evaluation on children. It's not that I don't think children are affected by stress; it's clear from conditions such as enuresis (bedwetting) that they are and I will discuss briefly the kinds of things parents might do to recognize when stress is a factor and how they might respond.

However, for reasons that are unclear, cortisol tests from children rarely provide conclusive results. Consequently, if I complete a food intolerance evaluation and symptoms persist, I move on to evaluating toxic load. If the problems still have not resolved, I skip the age management evaluation (for obvious reasons) and move to allopathic options.

THREE STEPS INSTEAD OF FIVE

Like the adult algorithm, Dr. Jheeta's Algorithm for children begins with body composition. For children and adolescents, I use the classic BMI adapted to children's bodies. The adult method of measuring waist-to-chest or waist-to-hips ratios does not work for prepubescent children for obvious reasons, and with adolescents it's difficult to know when their bodies have finished growing.

Consequently, to check children's body composition I use the standard BMI adapted for children. That is, I calculate the BMI and then compare it to standardized growth charts to determine where your child's body composition falls. I will provide more information on how you can check your child's BMI in Chapter 25. My main message here is that children need to be aware of their body composition, just as adults do. They should not eat indiscriminately, any more than adults should. They should learn to eat healthy nutritious food in appropriate portions from a young age.

As with adults, the next stage of the algorithm for children is testing for food intolerances. Children's intestines may not be fully colonized with the right gut flora until they're three-years-old. This makes them particularly susceptible during the early years of life to developing intolerances that could remain with them, unidentified, for an unknown period of time. Testing for food intolerances early can help to heal any damage done by introducing the wrong types of foods to developing digestive systems.

In the children's version of the algorithm, I move directly from testing for food intolerances to testing for toxic load. Children's developing bodies can make them susceptible to toxic exposure at lower levels. Allopathic doctors, too, take toxic exposure, even at low levels, in children very seriously as the consequences for neurological development can be severe and lifelong. I test for toxic load in children in exactly the same way as in adults. I also use the same treatment protocols.

Wellness testing does not apply to children, as it is really only intended for people over the age of 40. So if I've worked through body composition, food intolerances, and toxic load with a child without adequate symptomatic relief, I may recommend that the parent take the child to an allopathic physician to pursue further investigations.

This does not have to mean the end of my involvement. Allopathic treatments, while effective, can be harsh, and there may be supplements or therapies I can prescribe that will help keep the child's body strong to fight the effects of disease and of any allopathic therapies necessary to treat them. I am always happy to work with allopathic physicians in the best interest of any patient, but I find it particularly gratifying to work with children and help them learn first-hand about Generational Health First.

CHAPTER 18:
SPECIALIZED HEALTH CARE

It is very rare for a patient to leave my clinic having experienced no benefit whatsoever. When I speak of benefits, I mean objective measures such as weight lost, food intolerances identified, cortisol levels stabilized, lead levels reduced, or hormonal levels elevated. I also mean subjective benefits, from the patient's perspective, such as fulfilling a lifelong dream to go backpacking in Europe, getting back onto the tennis court and winning, or bringing a child in for evaluation 20 years after naturopathic care helped the parent when she was a child.

However, if a patient is 40 years or older, has worked through all five levels of Dr. Jheeta's Algorithm and is still experiencing significant health concerns, my next step is to discuss incorporating allopathic treatments in the care plan. This could include prescription drugs (naturopathic doctors in many areas now include an extensive list of prescription drugs in our scope of practice). It could mean working with an allopathic doctor to coordinate a treatment plan. Or, it could mean transferring care to an allopathic doctor, if that is in the patient's best interest.

Similarly, if I've worked through the first four levels of the algorithm with a patient who is under 40 without completely resolving symptoms, or if I've worked through the three levels of the algorithm for children without completely resolving a child's symptoms, I will move directly from treating for toxic load to an option that includes allopathic care.

As practicing physicians, naturopathic doctors understand the complex factors that contribute to various disease processes. Dr. Jheeta's Algorithm will never resolve every patient's health concerns. Effective referral is an important aspect of practicing medicine, and modern science has made a multi-disciplinary approach to healing more realistic than ever before in history.

Diagnosis and treatment of specific health problems is the crux of allopathic medicine. Nothing any alternative healing mode has to offer comes close to allopathic care for people who are injured or stricken with a communicable disease, or whose chronic degenerative disease processes have progressed past the point of prevention. Often, at these times, the best thing a naturopath can do is provide support for a patient's overall health while they fight the adverse effects of drugs and surgeries after all other courses of treatment have failed.

But even if a patient moves away from naturopathic care entirely, I always know their health has benefitted from working through my algorithm. These improvements will inevitably help them manage the health challenges they face. As more people take back control of their health, the well-being of the health-care system will improve, too, ensuring that, when a rare few patients must take extreme health measures, they will have the quickest and easiest possible access to this process.

PART III: EMPOWERMENT

INTRODUCTION

The tests I perform at each level of Dr. Jheeta's Algorithm are simple; the power lies in understanding the results. This understanding provides knowledge you may not have had in the past, enabling you to take action in the present, and produce real and lasting results in the future. It empowers you to change the way you think about your health and avoid preventable and potentially devastating consequences of poor health choices.

The first step to making changes of any kind is changing your point of view. It can be difficult to change a point of view you learned as a child from your parents and schools, and maintained into adult life along with your peers and with constant input from corporations and media. With information coming at you from every direction, it may never have occurred to you to question the sources you've always trusted.

But, if you are to truly look after yourself and your family, you sometimes have to question things. You have to ask whether you agree with all you've been taught and you have to open your mind to new ideas. I am not suggesting you indulge in trends just because their new and clever advertising campaigns make persuasive arguments. I'm only saying it's your responsibility as an individual to consider new ideas and work with those you decide are best for you and your family.

In this third and final section of the book, Empowerment, I will discuss the steps you can take to improve your health. I will walk you through things you can do to work through Dr. Jheeta's Algorithm, at first, with your naturopathic doctor, and then eventually on your own. In the back of the book, you'll find a list of research sources I've used in every chapter, most of them online and readily available for you to explore. As you follow the steps, think about using those resources to begin making this knowledge your own by researching it further. This type of information will give you the confidence you need to take back control of your health.

If by now you have decided to make changes to your health, I would recommend you start this with a naturopathic doctor to work with from the beginning. The Empowerment section of this book is here to help you understand what your naturopathic doctor is doing, and why. You can even use this part of the book to assess whether the naturopathic doctor you're considering is the right one for you, or is even qualified to be your doctor.

In Chapter 23, I've included information on how to find a good naturopathic doctor and know that he or she is fully qualified to meet your needs. Naturopathic medicine is still a young discipline and there are people in practice who claim to have proper naturopathic training, but do not. If you plan to work with a naturopathic doctor from the start, it's important to know what to look for and to avoid working with anyone who has not been properly trained at an accredited institution of naturopathic medicine. In a sense, this is another way of providing informed consent, and in writing Chapter 23, I felt this was some of the most empowering information I could provide.

Whether you decide to work through as much as possible of Dr. Jheeta's Algorithm on your own or seek professional help from the beginning, Part III will empower you to build awareness of the factors that influence your health, learn the questions to ask a health care provider, assess the answers you receive, and understand what you can do on your own, and what a naturopathic doctor can do to help you respond to your body's health challenges. That's what empowerment is all about.

CHAPTER 19:
TAKE CONTROL OF BODY COMPOSITION

I recently had a patient in his early forties. He came to me with concerns after a routine check-up with his family doctor showed he was hypertensive, had high cholesterol, and borderline high blood sugar.

"Tell me about yourself," I said on his first visit. "Do you smoke or drink? Do you get much exercise? Have you ever been hospitalized?"

"I don't smoke," he said. "I only drink on the weekends, and then mostly beer. I've never been really sick or needed surgery. I'm a trucker, he said, so I spend a lot of time sitting. I work out occasionally, but I'm pretty strong so it's not a regular thing."

"What about your family background," I asked.

"I'm from a large family—three sisters, two brothers. I grew up on the prairies. No major medical issues in my family."

We started working through phase one of the algorithm. His was a classic case of poor body composition. His waist measurement was significantly larger than his chest. When I reviewed his diet, I quickly realized he had no awareness of the idea of food portioning.

"How do you decide how much to eat at each meal?" I asked.

"I eat until I'm full," he said. "Is there something wrong with that?"

"If you always eat until you're full," I said, "you're eating to grow. As you grow, it takes more and more food to fill you up. So you keep eating more, and you keep getting bigger."

I didn't ask, but I suspected as a child, he'd been told to eat until his "plate was clean." Parents often say this for various reasons, but if we eat according to the amount on our plates, we don't learn to pay attention to how our bodies feel.

"Learning good food portioning can help you achieve and maintain a good weight," I said to him. "That depends on the amount of physical activity you do – calories in for calories out. You need to learn to estimate portion size by sight, eat it slowly, and then stop. You also need to choose high-impact foods rather than empty calories."

"I don't know what you mean by 'food portioning,' 'high-impact food,' and 'empty calories,'" he said. "I've always thought food was food."

"Are you open to learning a different way of looking at things?" I asked.

"Well, that's why I'm here," he said. "So I guess I am."

Once he understood these basic principles, we developed a regular, moderate exercise routine he could maintain permanently – nothing extreme. The issue for him wasn't to build strength but to lose weight, keep it off, and get his blood pressure, blood sugar, and cholesterol under control. The idea was to set realistic exercise goals so he wouldn't dread working out and find excuses not to do it.

With the basic building blocks in place, we established two goals: a 500-calorie per day reduction in intake and a 400-calorie per day increase in exercise. With a net reduction of 900 calories per day, we planned for him to drop two to four pounds per month. After a year, he'd lost 50 pounds, his blood parameters were normal, and there was no reason to continue beyond the first level of the algorithm.

TAKE BACK CONTROL ONE STEP AT A TIME

In the evaluation section, I talked about the direct correlation between body composition and risk of heart disease, diabetes, and other chronic diseases. Some of my patients resolve all their health issues by simply taking control of their body composition.

In this chapter, you will start acting on this knowledge by doing the measurements. Remember, if you're a man, your chest should be larger than your waist, even if only by an inch. If you're a woman, your hips should be larger than your waist, even if only by an inch. This provides plenty of room for variation in body size and type.

If your measurements are not within this range, you will need to make changes. If you feel your weight issues are related to metabolism, have this checked out by your ND/NMD or MD, but for 90% of the patients I see, this is not the case.

THE PLAIN TRUTH: MOST OF US EAT TOO MUCH!

If your measurements reveal your body composition is not what it should be, look closely at your diet and ask a few questions:

- What am I eating?
- How much am I eating?
- When am I eating?
- Why am I eating?

Most of us eat the wrong things, we eat too much of everything, we eat at the wrong times of day, we eat for fun instead of fuel, and we don't burn off what we eat with physical activity. Our food is controlling us instead of us controlling our relationship with food. We are eating ourselves to death.

One way to begin taking back control is with a food diary. A food diary can help you be more conscious about what you eat. When you write everything down, you can't eat absentmindedly. Also, surveying your eating habits as you look back over your diary can help you identify triggers – moments or situations when you tend to eat, like when you're under stress, or at a party – and develop healthier coping mechanisms.

According to *WebMD*, "Several studies have shown that people who keep food journals are more likely to be successful in losing weight and keeping it off. In fact, a researcher from one recent study says that people keeping a food diary six days a week lost about twice as much weight as those who kept food records one day a week or less."[*]

TAKE CONTROL OF *WHAT* YOU EAT

Let's start with what you shouldn't eat. As a rule, avoid any food advertised on TV. Occasionally, associations that represent farmers

---

[*] "Can a Food Diary Help You Lose Weight?" by Elaine Magee, *WebMD*, http://www.webmd.com/diet/features/can-food-diary-help-you-lose-weight.

advertise eggs, milk, blueberries, or other farm products on TV. These are not my concerns. The point is to eat whole, unprocessed foods as much as possible.

It's okay to eat some processed foods, but try not to make them daily choices, and try to choose those that have been processed as little as possible. For example, having frozen vegetables on your plate a couple of times a week is not a problem, as long as you eat fresh vegetables on other days. If you crave something sweet after dinner, why not enjoy a dish of canned fruit (preferably packed in fruit juice without added sugar and packaged in a glass jar rather than a tin). The main points are to:

- Avoid heavily processed foods, like white pasta in a box with powdered sauces, frozen meals you heat up in the microwave, or packaged desserts heavy with refined sugar and processed fats.
- Limit how often you eat fat-laden burgers, fries, and other fast foods.
- Avoid munching on sweets, potato chips, and other snack foods.

Remember salt, sugar and fat are not what real fruits and vegetables taste like! Once you begin cutting out processed foods and rediscovering what real food tastes like, you might find there's a whole world of food you didn't even know existed.

Okay, so that's what I shouldn't do. Now what should I do?

The key things are to incorporate some protein (meat, fish, eggs, cheese, beans, nuts), produce (fresh fruit and vegetables), and whole grains (whole wheat, whole spelt, quinoa, millet, brown rice) into every meal. Whole grains and protein take time to break down, so they stave off hunger longer. Fruits and vegetables are loaded with antioxidants, which helps your body fight things like plaque build-up in your arteries.

Also be sure to eat foods with fibre (like whole grains) to keep food moving through your digestive system. As I've discussed, food that gets backed up in your intestines can lead to a number of issues including leaky gut syndrome. This is why I would like to see everyone re-learn what food taste like in it's original state, fruits and vegetables for example, instead of relying on a pre-programmed addiction to manufactured tastes that include salts, refined sugars, and saturated fats. Here are some suggestions to help you get started. See "Your Daily Diet" chart on page 141 for some healthy do's and don'ts.

YOUR DAILY DIET

	Do	Don't
Breakfast	**Do** choose whole-grain toast, or cereals such as oatmeal. **Do** have some protein, like eggs, cheese, or nuts. **Do** munch on a bit of fruit or a drink a small glass of fruit juice.	**Don't** start your day with doughnuts, muffins, or other sweet pastries, or "instant" breakfast beverages. **Don't** skip breakfast, or have only coffee.
Lunch	**Do** make a sandwich with whole-grain bread. **Do** enjoy a hearty bowl of soup **Do** chomp on some raw vegetables or a salad, easy on the dressing. **Do** include protein in your meal.	**Don't** scarf down a cheeseburger and fries, or other greasy fried food. **Don't** have pop or chips with your meal. **Don't** skip lunch, or have only a chocolate bar or muffin.

Supper	Do grill, bake, or broil meat. Do fill your plate half full with vegetables, one-quarter full with starch, and one-quarter full with protein. Do enjoy a dish of canned fruit or applesauce for dessert.	Don't fry meat, potatoes, or vegetables. Don't smother foods in fatty gravies, sauces, and condiments. Don't top your meal off with pies, cakes, and cookies.
Snacks	Do choose a piece of fruit, some fresh vegetables with a yogurt dip, or a handful of nuts.	Don't snack on potato chips, chocolate bars, or other junk foods between meals.

TAKE CONTROL OF *HOW MUCH* YOU EAT

If I suggested you cut 500 calories per day from your diet, would you know how?

Um – maybe?

That's fine, because counting calories and watching pounds every day is not the best way to lose weight. It's fine to set a weekly time to weigh yourself, and to have a good general idea of the caloric value of various foods. But when you count every calorie, it's easy to become over-focused on squeezing in every allowable bit instead of noticing how your food makes you feel. Also, it's not always possible to know how many calories are in every dish prepared in a restaurant or at someone else's home, which makes it easier to kid yourself into thinking you've eaten fewer calories than you really have.

What's a better way?

Learn to judge portion sizes by the way they look, and adjust food intake by paying attention to the way you feel. There are several tricks for reducing portion sizes. One is to buy smaller dinner plates so it takes less food to fill your plate. Another is to serve up what you would normally have, and then put 25% back. A third is to fill your plate half full with vegetables, and divide the other half equally between protein (meat, fish, eggs, cheese, beans) and carbohydrates (potatoes, grains, pasta).

You can find many more tricks for reducing and managing food intake on the Internet. Here are a few examples:

- Drink a glass of cool water 10-15 minutes before a meal; you will feel full sooner and eat less.
- Take small bites and chew thoroughly; you will enjoy your food more, and start the digestive process in a healthier way.
- Wait five minutes (or even two or three) before going back for seconds or dessert; by that time, you'll probably realize you've had enough.
- Only eat at a table; this helps shed habits like eating junk food while working or watching TV, or wolfing food down on the run.
- Eat with others whenever possible; eating with family provides time to keep up with loved one's lives, and provides a chance to role model good habits for children. Numerous studies suggest children who share meals with their families have healthier diets as adults.

TAKE CONTROL OF *WHEN* YOU EAT

One of the best weight-loss strategies is to eat breakfast. Patients often tell me they skip breakfast because they're too busy, too tired to get up early enough to eat, or trying to lose weight and don't want the extra calories. But, eating breakfast provides energy to keep up with busy schedules, get through the day's tasks, and get to sleep without feeling stressed. When you skip breakfast, you're more likely to snack between meals and overeat at meals to compensate for starting your day off hungry.

The important thing about breakfast is to avoid marketing traps. Food companies know people are pressed for time, and often say a breakfast beverage, instant cereal, or breakfast bar can provide the nutrition to start the day right, but virtually all "instant" breakfast foods are heavily processed and high in sugar; even instant oatmeal has the same effect as refined sugar when it hits your blood stream. When that happens, you get a sugar spike followed by a sugar crash. By lunch time, you're ravenous and you spend your day eating the same way as if you'd skipped breakfast. That "instant" breakfast has set you up for a day of overeating.

The best way to start your day, especially if you're watching your weight, is with a healthy breakfast. It's even more important for parents to role model this for children. The American Dietetic Association tells us that "children who eat breakfast perform better in the classroom and on the playground, with better concentration, problem-solving skills, and eye-hand coordination..."[†]

But what is there to eat for breakfast since eggs have become a big no-no?

Eggs are NOT a no-no. Eggs got a bad rap during the low-fat campaign. For years, more than three eggs a week were thought to increase cholesterol, but that was before researchers understood the differences between good and bad fats. In the same article as quoted above, *WebMD* describes a study that compared weight loss in women who ate either two eggs or a bagel for breakfast:

> *Compared to the bagel eaters, overweight women who ate two eggs for breakfast five times a week for eight weeks as part of a low-fat, reduced-calorie diet, lost 65% more weight, reduced waist circumference by 83%, reported higher energy levels, and had no significant difference in their...blood cholesterol or triglyceride levels.*

So taking control of when you eat is all about eating a healthy breakfast?

Yes and no. Starting the day out right seems to put us on the right track toward eating at meal times and not snacking in between. There are many other factors, but they often have less to do with what or when we eat than why we eat.

[†] "The Many Benefits of Breakfast," by Kathleen M. Zelman, *WebMD*, http://www.webmd.com/diet/features/many-benefits-breakfast.

TAKE CONTROL OF *WHY* YOU EAT

I often come back to Hippocrates' advice to "Let food be your medicine." But if good food can be good medicine, and bad food or too much food can be bad medicine, then eating any food beyond your needs for fuel can also be bad medicine.

But you said eating with others is good, and we don't always eat with others to provide our bodies with energy. Sometimes, it's more about socializing than refuelling, isn't it?

There's a difference between using our common need to refuel as an opportunity to spend time with friends and family, and using friends and family as an excuse to eat. If you're in the habit of eating beyond your fuel needs, you'll find many reasons to eat, like alleviating stress, munching on junk food while you watch TV, or using alcohol as a social lubricant.

Those kinds of eating habits can be the hardest to break, which is why it's so important to instil good eating habits in your children. I've seen patients try for years to break or change poor eating habits they learned when they were young. It's futile to tell people to stop eating when deep-seated social and emotional triggers control their urges.

In the clinic, we have counselling to help patients assess their eating habits. Once they understand why they're eating, they can move forward, slowly incorporating new foods and new ways of handling triggers. If you're trying to do this on your own, the first step is to notice when you eat, what you eat, how much you eat, and why you eat – your food diary is ideal for that.

Okay, but writing down every chip I eat at a party could be awkward.

That's partly the point. Many people report that making the commitment to write everything down often discourages them from snacking. It isn't worth the trouble, and it also makes them more conscious about how often they eat mindlessly. One problem with this type of eating is that you can be overweight, yet suffering from malnutrition.

Malnutrition! How's that possible?

148

I remember a friend-of-a-friend story about a woman in her forties who'd tried to lose weight for years. She'd skip meals, work out like crazy, and lose lots of weight quickly, but then put it all back on again, and gain even more. She was completely frustrated, until she sought nutritional counselling.

The first steps were blood tests and a food journal. When the nutrition counsellor saw the journal, she began asking questions. It came out that the patient had had a complicated childhood. Every time things got crazy around her house, she ate. As an adult, every time she got stressed, she ate. She'd gain weight, and then starve herself, work out for two hours daily, and lose the weight. But, that wasn't sustainable, so she'd stop working out, go back to eating empty calories, and regain the weight all over again.

When she first sought help, she was 50 pounds overweight, yet malnourished. Once she stopped skipping meals, started eating a balanced diet, and reduced her workouts to a sustainable routine, she lost 50 pounds and kept it off.

She reduced her workouts?

Yes and no. Instead of working out for two hours every night for two months, until she was too exhausted to continue, and then getting no exercise at all for six months, she began working out for one-hour, three times a week, which she could sustain. It took about a year and a lot of hard work but, just like the man at the beginning of this chapter, she took back control of her body composition, and probably reduced her risk for many chronic diseases at the same time. Perhaps without thinking about it, she chose prevention over palliation.

TAKING BACK CONTROL TAKES TIME

Losing weight takes time. We often see patients who complain they have put on 20 pounds in a year but don't want to accept that it may take just as long to lose the weight. Often patients undertake extreme diets in an effort to lose 20 pounds in a month. That's possible, but not a good idea.

Diets of fewer than about 1,100 calories per day carry extreme health risks. The first few pounds you lose are water, which you can quickly regain. If you continue dieting, your body will start burning fat, but it will also start burning muscle, which can cause dizziness, confusion, fatigue, and intolerance to cold. If you continue an extreme diet, you'll shortchange your body on vitamins and minerals, which may be why the woman I talked about was malnourished.

Extreme dieting can even cause heart attack and death. If you're old enough to remember a rock group from the 1960s called The Mamas & the Papas, you may remember that's how "Mama" Cass Elliott died. Karen Carpenter, a singer from the 1970s group, The Carpenters, had a different eating disorder (she was anorexic and bulimic, but the emotional causes of many eating disorders can be similar), but, like Elliott, she died of heart failure.

That's tragic. But are you saying that if I want to lose 40 pounds without endangering my health, I can expect to be on a diet for two years?

No. The healthiest rate for weight loss is one to two pounds per week, which means you can safely lose 40 pounds in 20 weeks. But rather than going on a diet, which research has repeatedly shown doesn't work, you have to develop healthy and sustainable eating and lifestyle habits. Once you reach your goal weight, you may add a few calories daily or ease up a bit on your workouts, but your plan should be to make lasting changes, such as working out regularly, learning healthy food portioning, and cutting out junk food.

If your diet has included a lot of junk food and fast food for many years you may need to experiment to find the best way to "kick the junk food habit." Remember, processed sugar, fat, and salt have many of the same addictive properties as hard drugs. While some people find it easiest to go cold turkey (stop consuming the addictive substance and get through the symptoms of withdrawal all at once), others prefer to go more slowly.

For example, say your food diary shows you eat some kind of junky snack food five times a day: morning coffee break, after lunch, afternoon coffee break, after supper, and while watching TV in the evening. So, the first week, you substitute a piece of fruit or a dish of yogurt during your morning break. The second week, you substitute a healthier option after lunch, too.

Do you mean, make changes gradually?

Yes. And don't beat yourself up if you have some failures. Mistakes and failures are actually good, because they help you learn what you need to succeed, and what undermines your efforts. Do you prefer to wade into cold water slowly, or would you rather jump off the pier in one big splash? When you learn what you need to be successful at weight loss, or any other goal, you will probably also learn about what you need to be successful in other areas of your life.

It sounds like you're saying people should accept themselves as they are, but doesn't that contradict what you're saying about needing to change?

No. I'm saying people come in all shapes and sizes, some of which are genetically determined. If you're a woman with ample hips but you know you're eating right and exercising enough, celebrate your curves! If you're a man who's short and muscular but you're satisfied with your caloric intake and output, consider yourself compact!

Your goal should be to accept your basic shape and personality as they are, but recognize what you can change physically, and learn to use your personality traits to help you make those changes. I'm always in favour of people doing what they can to maximize their health, but the last thing I want is for anyone to develop disordered eating or exercise habits because they've set unrealistic goals that will never fit their body type or personality.

Focus on your health. Think about your health habits and their possible consequences in the future. You may be able to get away with bad habits now, but eventually the impacts of those habits will catch up to you. Without knowing you and your family history, I can't say whether the consequences are likely to be diabetes, arthritis, heart disease, cancer, or any other debilitating degenerative disease that could have horrific consequences for you and those who love you, but if do something about it now, you can reduce your own risk while setting a positive example for your children and other loved ones.

GET MOVING!

As I mentioned earlier, it's only in the last 70 years that researchers have begun to look specifically at the connection between exercise, or lack of it, and development of chronic disease. Up until then, perhaps because most people got physical exercise in the course of their daily lives, no one had connected the dots between physical activity and health.

There are three basic types of exercise, and each one plays a role in helping you take back control of your health and decrease your risk of chronic ill health. Those three types are:

- Aerobic or cardiovascular exercise, which uses large muscle groups and builds heart-lung capacity;
- Anaerobic exercise or resistance training, which strengthens specific muscle groups;
- Flexibility training, which stretches and lengthens muscle groups and increases joint flexibility.

GET YOUR HEART PUMPING

Cardiovascular (CV) exercise can include running, bicycling, swimming, dancing, skating, and so on, but you can also get a CV workout simply by walking quickly. Whatever you do to get your heart pumping faster and your lungs working harder is CV exercise. This offers many benefits to body composition:

- It's the best way to burn calories, which can help you lose weight and keep it off. You have to burn off as many calories as you take in to maintain weight – more if you want to lose weight.
- It's the best way to burn off cortisol. Cortisol increases blood sugar to make more energy available in stressful situations, but if you don't burn off blood sugar with physical exercise, it turns to fat. So CV exercise can prevent you from gaining weight under stress.
- It builds the size and strength of your heart. Your heart is the strongest muscle in your body, and needs to be exercised to withstand stress and strain. Also, as your heart gets stronger,

152

your metabolism quickens, allowing your body to burn more calories even when you are at rest.

CV exercise also increases levels of HDL (good) cholesterol in your body, while decreasing unhealthy fats and reducing risk of heart disease, stroke, diabetes, arthritis, and even cancer. CV exercise stimulates production of brain chemicals that improve mood and self-esteem. Because of its effect on your metabolism, CV exercise makes you feel energetic. If your CV workout includes weight-bearing exercise, such as running or walking, it helps build bone density and provide protection against osteoporosis. All types of CV exercise build muscle, but some ways of working out, such as swimming and rowing, build many major muscle groups simultaneously.

There are many different schools of thought on how to get CV exercise. Raising your heart rate from its resting rate (beats per minute when lying down) to training zone (beats per minute during exercise, calculated on the basis of age) and keeping it there for at least 20 minutes three to four times weekly has long been considered the best way to keep your heart strong and healthy.

If you haven't been getting regular CV exercise for a while, start small and build. Go for a 10-minute walk every day (maybe give yourself one day a week off). Walk quickly enough that you can feel yourself breathing more heavily than usual, but not so quickly that you can't have a conversation with a friend walking with you. Add five minutes per week to your walk until you're up to at least 30 minutes.

If you can't manage a 30-minute workout every day, elevate your heart rate for as many accumulated minutes over the day as you can manage, even if it's in five-minute bursts. Any exercise is better than no exercise, so if one longer walk daily doesn't fit your schedule, try two 5-minute walks, and later add a third, and maybe a fourth. Do whatever works for you, because if it doesn't work for you, you won't do it, and that won't do you any good at all.

BUILD YOUR MUSCLE STRENGTH

Strength training has many of the same benefits as CV training, but rather than developing heart and lung capacity, it builds lean muscle mass. Here's why lean muscle mass is a good thing:

- It burns more calories than fatty tissue does;
- It helps you endure stress and strain without injury;
- It reduces discomfort and symptoms associated with chronic back pain, arthritis, obesity, heart disease, and diabetes;
- It helps with balance and reduces risk of falls.**

**If you're young and healthy, you may think falling is not a big deal, but falls are a major cause of injury at every age, and can be particularly problematic among older people, sometimes forcing them to give up their independence long before they want to. If you want to remain independent for as long as possible, stay strong now!

According to the Harvard Public School of Health, strength training is probably the most neglected aspect of fitness but one of the most important. "In fact, it's so beneficial that the American College of Sports Medicine, the American Heart Association, and the 2008 Physical Activity Guidelines for Americans recommend that adults engage in strength training at least twice a week, to improve muscle strength and endurance."‡

There are many different approaches to strength training. You can go to a gym and ask the staff to help work out a routine that will fit for you, with resistance machines or free weights, or you can do resistance training at home at little to no cost. Resistance tubing, for example, is inexpensive and can provide excellent strength training simply by holding it in two hands or wrapping it around the feet or legs and pulling in opposite directions. Or you can use your own body weight to build muscle through push-ups, sit-ups, abdominal crunches, leg squats, and leg raises – the ways you can use your own body to build muscle strength are almost limitless.

As with CV training, the key is to start small and build. For the first week, you might do five push-ups, five sit-ups, five leg

---

‡ "Strength and Flexibility Training," *The Nutrition Source,* Harvard School of Public Health, http://www.hsph.harvard.edu/nutritionsource/strength-and-flexibility-training/.

squats, and five leg raises on each side. If that's too much, try modified exercises, such as knee or wall push-ups or partial sit-ups. Each week, increase the number of *reps* (repetitions) of each exercise. Or, when you're ready, increase the challenge level by trading your first five wall push-ups for knee push-ups, or your first five partial sits for full sit-ups.

Whatever approach you choose: take it slowly. If you move too quickly, you could cause an injury, and then you'll need to take time off to heal. That would be a setback. Remember, the goal is to build strength gradually, not hurt yourself.

INCREASE YOUR FLEXIBILITY

A website called *Sport Fitness Advisor* defines flexibility "as the range of motion about a joint and its surrounding muscles during a passive movement." Increasing range of motion can enhance performance and reduce risk of injury. "The rationale for this is that a limb can move further before an injury occurs."[8]

It's an interesting theory, though the idea that flexibility training can prevent injury is still being debated. However, the importance of flexibility in helping adults maintain range of motion is well accepted. Again quoting the Harvard Public School of Health, "the American Heart Association recommends that healthy adults engage in flexibility training two to three days per week, stretching major muscle and tendon groups," though some schools of thought suggest that older adults reduce this to twice weekly.

There are too many different ways to use flexibility training to improve range of motion to describe here. Key points are to:

- Stretch when you muscles are warm, such as after your CV workout;
- Move slowly into the desired stretch, and then hold for 15 to 60 seconds;
- Don't bounce and don't lock your joints, as you hold, you should be able to feel your muscles loosening up and realize that you are able to settle a little further into the stretch;

[8] "The Benefits of Flexibility Training," Flexibility Training Section, *Sports Fitness Advisor,* http://www.sport-fitness-advisor.com/flexibilitytraining.html.

- Remember to breathe while you're stretching;
- Repeat each stretch at least four times.

In the Sources section at the back of the book, you will find a link to a "Sample Flexibility Plan for Beginners," which provides descriptions and photos of many stretches. As with other types of exercise, the important thing is to start small and build. Too many people sit at desks all day, developing neck and back pain, repetitive strain injury, and stiff joints. Many books, magazine articles, and websites can help you start with simple exercises you can perform at your desk or while watching television. The important thing is to start sooner rather than later.

ENJOY YOUR EXERCISE

Exercise is inherently repetitive and can be boring, so you need to find ways to keep it interesting and fun. Many years ago, a woman I know used to meet a friend at a bus stop to go for a swim in the university pool before classes started. Often they would get to the bus stop and one would say, "I wouldn't be here if I didn't know you were here waiting for me." Then the other one would laugh and say, "I only came for you!" But by that time, they were there, so they'd go for their morning swim and feel good all day for having done it.

Exercising with a friend is one way to stay motivated, but even if you prefer to exercise alone, there are ways to keep yourself on track. Most importantly, do exercise that you enjoy. There's no point in planning to go the gym three days a week if you really hate the gym and won't ever go.

If that's the case, find something you might like better. Do you enjoy team sports? Investigate a local league for volleyball, basketball, or hockey. Do you love the outdoors? Look into hiking, kayaking, or skiing. Want something that will help you find calm in the middle of a hectic day? Join a yoga class or try a martial art.

Once you've found a type of exercise you like, figure out what time of day works best for you. Some people like to start their day with a morning run or a bike ride to work; others prefer to sweat off their stress at the gym or in a kickboxing class on the way home from work.

If you feel like you're not getting anywhere, try tracking your progress in an exercise journal.

You've talked about a food diary for weight loss, but what's an exercise journal?

It's very similar to a food diary, but you use it to record information like when you worked out, for how long, what type of exercise you did, how many reps, and any other details that you can use as markers of your progress. Every so often, look back at where you were three or six months earlier to see how far you've come.

I often have a hard time sticking it out with exercise because I get bored.

Exercise can be tedious and repetitious, but there are so many different ways to enjoy physical activity that there's really no reason to get bored. Try doing two or three different types of workouts in a week. Perhaps go the gym twice, go for a swim twice, and one day a week go for a long walk. Again, the important thing is to accept yourself as you are, not as an excuse for not exercising, but to figure out what works best for you.

MOVE FORWARD

Typically, after six to eight weeks of dietary changes that reduce caloric intake by 200–500 per day, paired with building up to moderate exercise for 30 minutes per day, five days per week, most of my patients have already begun improving their body composition and resolving their symptoms. Sometimes, improving body composition is all my patients have to do to reduce their risk of chronic degenerative disease. However, if, at this point a patient is still experiencing symptoms, I urge them to continue taking responsibility for their health by exploring food intolerances.

CHAPTER 20:
TAKE CONTROL OF FOOD
INTOLERANCES

An acquaintance of mine has Crohn's disease (she is the mother of the girl I mentioned in Chapter 1). As a young woman, it forced her to cut back on a lot of the foods she ate, but she gradually got most of them back and for many years ate a normal diet and lived a normal life.

Years passed, until one day, when she was enjoying her favourite treat – an iced latté – she noticed it was causing abdominal pain. It wasn't the first time; she'd been feeling bloated off and on for a while. But that day, she realized she couldn't ignore it any longer and made an appointment with her allopathic doctor.

"A colonoscopy a few months later gave me the good news, she says. My Crohn's disease was not active and I wouldn't need surgery, but it also gave me the bad news: the scar tissue left by the Crohn's was causing irritable bowel syndrome (IBS) and the only way to control it was to go back to the tedious process of identifying problem foods and avoiding them. I dreaded it," she said.

Food is a central part of our lives. In a culture that offers up fancy coffees, drinks at the bar, and parties with cheese trays and sweet treats, it can be hard to feel included when there's so much you can't enjoy with everyone else.

"Coffee was the first thing to go," she says. " – And the hardest. I didn't realize how addicted I was until I tried to give it up. I'd stop drinking it and feel better. So I'd decide I could just have it occasionally and slip back into having it every day. But then all the symptoms would come back.

It took me between five and ten years to get off it for good," she says. "But once I did, I felt so much better. Getting off coffee gave me the impetus to start tackling other problem foods: wheat, dairy, alcohol. Once I was off coffee, I realized how much it was increasing my sensitivity to other foods and work out how often I could indulge in some of my sensitivities without the same ill effects. At that point, I finally stopped dreading the process and started embracing it, because I knew in the end I'd feel better."

Or to put it another way, she was taking back control of her health.

EMPOWERMENT WITH CAUTION

As I said earlier, my view, as naturopathic doctor, is that all food intolerances occur on a spectrum. At one end of the spectrum is mild sensitivity, which causes some discomfort, usually in the digestive tract. At the other end is anaphylaxis, a full-on immune system offensive which, in its effort to expel something the body wrongly perceives as a dangerous invader, can cause such severe swelling of the airways as to cut off oxygen to the brain, and cause brain damage or even death.

Most food intolerances cause symptoms somewhere between these two extremes. The symptoms are often, but not always, digestive in nature, ranging from mild to extremely uncomfortable. In this chapter, I'll focus on taking control of food intolerances by learning how to identify foods that are causing problems, and what to do then.

First, however, as a responsible naturopathic physician, I need to caution you against self-diagnosing food intolerances at the anaphylactic end of the spectrum. This is why everyone starting the process of using my algorithm should see a naturopathic physician to get started on the path to testing, and diagnosis.

Almost all anaphylactic reactions are discovered by accident. A person must have been exposed to an allergen (offending substance) at least once for the immune system to develop an anaphylactic response. Anaphylactic reactions typically escalate with each subsequent exposure. Usually within the first two or three exposures, the patient will need emergency measures, the doctor will note the symptoms and severity, and diagnose anaphylaxis. Then the doctor will advise the patient to avoid the allergen completely, wear a medical alert ID bracelet, and carry an Epipen (single-dose injection of epinephrine) and antihistamines (such as Benadryl) at all times.

No qualified naturopathic doctor will test for an anaphylactic response. The implications of inducing anaphylaxis are too dangerous. Any qualified naturopathic doctor is prepared to handle in-office anaphylaxis with an adrenaline shot, oxygen, AED (a defibrillator to respond to cardiac arrest), and IV infusion, if necessary, but any qualified naturopathic doctor will agree the best way to deal with anaphylaxis is to prevent it by avoiding the problem food.

Is it possible to grow out of anaphylaxis?

It was once thought children diagnosed with anaphylaxis would never outgrow it, but in recent years allopathic allergy specialists have noticed that some adults have done just that. I know of a young man who was diagnosed in childhood with anaphylaxis to fish and seafood, but in adulthood has found he is able to eat fish, but not shellfish.

However, if you grew up with anaphylaxis and wonder if you have outgrown it, you should only have it tested under highly controlled conditions: usually first screened with a blood test, followed by a skin prick test in a doctor's office where all emergency measures are available.

Can people fail to realize they have anaphylaxis until they're adults?

It's unlikely. However, it is possible for adults to develop an anaphylactic response to a food they've previously consumed without problems. The most common food in this category is shellfish, but I've heard of adults developing reactions to other foods, such as eggs. Once adults develop such severe responses, it's unlikely they'll ever outgrow them.

If you think you or your child may have an anaphylactic allergy, do not try to diagnose it yourself. Seek professional help under controlled conditions and follow your doctor's advice exactly.

The foods most likely to trigger anaphylaxis are not all obvious. In Canada, these have been identified as: eggs, milk, mustard, peanuts, seafood (fish, crustaceans, and shellfish), sesame, soy, sulphites, tree nuts, and wheat. The list of the top eight in the US is similar: cow's milk, peanuts, shellfish, tree nuts, eggs, fish, soy, and wheat.

However, figuring out where these foods are hiding can be tricky, often many products have recipes containing some of the foods listed. Ask any parent of a child with anaphylaxis how quickly they became expert label readers, and how surprised they were to find where offending foods can hide, such as wheat in soy sauce and nuts in hand lotion.

THE USUAL SUSPECTS

Ideally, you would always have professional help to sort out food intolerances, but that's not always possible. Sometimes, you realize you don't feel right and don't know why. Maybe you wake up in the morning and feel fine, but soon after you start eating you feel bloated and you have abdominal cramps.

Maybe despite all the advice to start each day with a good breakfast, you avoid it because you're eating something that seems healthy but makes you feel bad. Or maybe there are days when you feel great all day, but out of the blue you start feeling "off" and don't know why. You explain it to your allopathic doctor, and he sends you for some tests, but the results all come back negative, yet you know you don't feel right.

Learning whether food intolerances are the root cause of your discomfort can be challenging. By the time your symptoms are bad enough for you to do something about them, the problems have been building for a while and it may take some effort to sort them out. One way to start is simply to learn which foods most commonly cause intolerant reactions.

As a naturopathic doctor, I'm not surprised by the amount of overlap between mild food sensitivities and anaphylactic responses (eggs, milk, mustard, peanuts, fish/seafood, sesame, soy, sulphites, tree nuts, and wheat). I don't think this is a coincidence; it supports the theory that all intolerances occur on a spectrum.

A British association called Allergy UK categorizes common intolerances a little differently:

- Alcohol intolerance is most often based on the food from which the alcohol is made (grapes, hops, barley) or other substances in the beverage (such as sulphites, yeasts, or histamine).
- Histamine intolerance can be triggered by high-histamine foods, including many alcoholic drinks, pickled foods, cheeses, mushrooms, yeast, and chocolate.
- Dairy intolerance is most often due to the milk sugar (lactose) in cow's milk, but can be triggered by milk protein. Some people who can't tolerate cow's milk can manage sheep or goat milk.
- Wheat and gluten intolerance are not the same thing. It's possible to be intolerant to gluten proteins (which are also present in grains such as rye and barley) rather than the wheat itself.
- Yeast intolerance can be difficult to diagnose because yeast is present in many foods. Bread is obvious, but yeast is also present in fermented foods, such as alcohol, vinegar, soy sauce, and ripe miso. Sometimes an apparent wheat, dairy, or alcohol intolerance is really yeast intolerance.

With all this overlap, it can be difficult to identify your food intolerances. Also, allergenic foods can be buried in small amounts inside other foods. Eggs, for example, are in many baked goods in such small quantities they're far down the ingredient list, but if you're strongly intolerant, you may still react. If you eat foods that don't contain nuts but are made in the same facility as nut-containing foods, you might react. If you are intolerant to gluten rather than wheat, you might not realize barley malt syrup (used as a sweetener) could cause the same symptoms.

Intolerances to sulphites or histamine can be even more difficult to diagnose: histamine is a chemical that occurs naturally in many foods, and sulphites are often used as preservatives, but neither of these allergens necessarily appear on any food label. You can also exacerbate intolerance reactions by eating two problem foods together, by eating a large quantity of the offending food, or by eating small quantities frequently. It's easy to tell patients to avoid any food that causes a problem, but with all these complications, it can be difficult to figure out which foods are causing problems.

TRACK INTOLERANCES WITH A FOOD DIARY

The first step I take in diagnosing food intolerances is a blood test, but you can't really do that for yourself at home. However, you can start by keeping a food diary. If you've already used a food diary for weight loss, you'll remember how it works. If you haven't, you use it to record when you ate, what you ate, and how much you ate. But, instead of recording why you ate, note how you felt before and after you ate.

You mean how I felt, physically, right? I'd want to know how I felt emotionally if I were trying to lose weight, but physically to diagnose food intolerances – right?

Actually, in this instance, you need to note both emotional and physical reactions. Remember, the mind-body works on a continuum. Some foods cause obvious symptoms, like gassiness and cramping, while others cause subtler reactions. One mom I know had been tracking her two-year-old's intolerances since he began having a projectile-vomit reaction to cow's milk when he was eight months old. One weekend when he was a toddler, out of nowhere, he began having five-hour temper tantrums that would only end when he fell asleep, exhausted.

After two or three of these tantrums, the mom realized something was not right and made a list of everything her son had eaten since the tantrums started. The only variation in his diet was a new brand of soymilk, sweetened with barley malt syrup, and barley-malt contains gluten. All of his marathon tantrums had occurred within 20 minutes of his drinking a bottle of soymilk. She threw it out, and the tantrums stopped.

So if I have a sudden marathon temper tantrum, I'll know what to blame!

I would hope adults would express symptoms differently than a toddler. However, you could feel inexplicably listless and lethargic, or bloated and uncomfortable, and not realize until you start tracking your symptoms that this always occurs within a few hours after eating a certain food.

Figuring that out could be quite a process.

That's why a blood test is a much easier starting point, but if that's not practical for you, you can combine a food diary with lists like those I've provided to isolate broad general trends. For example, maybe over the course of two weeks, you notice that you start sniffing and wheezing every time you eat cheese, drink wine, or eat bread. If you often have a cheeseburger, ham and cheese sandwich, or pizza for lunch, and routinely pour a glass of wine when you get home from work, you could be sniffing and wheezing so often it becomes hard to identify the allergen as histamine. By keeping track of what you consume and when you feel good and bad, and then comparing the related foods with a list of common intolerances, you can get some idea of what foods to start eliminating.

A PROCESS OF ELIMINATION

There are many ways to undertake an elimination diet. One celebrity doctor recommends an elaborate cleanse before reintroducing foods. A company website called Precision Nutrition outlines an extensive and thorough process. If you do your research, you'll likely find dozens of approaches. But I don't know if any of them will be any more effective than the simple approach I suggest:

- If you suspect a food of causing you problems, stop eating it for six weeks.
- Notice if the problems go away.
- After six weeks, start eating it again and notice if the problems come back.
- If problems return, don't eat it anymore.

After nearly 30 years in practice, I find this method as effective as any other and not hard for patients to adhere to. As you progress with this approach, you may be able to start fine tuning. For example, in the situation I described above, on the basis of your reactions to cheese, wine, and bread, you may have withdrawn all dairy products, alcohol, and wheat from your diet. You may feel better a lot of the time, until one day you have a nice, healthy stir-fry with mushrooms, tofu, and soy sauce, and you start sniffing and wheezing again!

Because mushrooms, tofu, and soy sauce all contain histamine, and so do cheese, wine, and bread. Did I get that right?

Yes. Most people have an enzyme in their bodies called diamine oxidase, which breaks down the histamine in foods. But if your body is low in histamine and you absorb it through foods or environmental allergens, you will experience typical symptoms of allergy.

This could mean the problems are not what you thought they were. You'll only find out by re-introducing foods without histamine, like non-cheese dairy products. If you have no symptoms, you might try a stir-fry with meat, vegetables, and a different sauce, and feel fine. If you eliminate all histamine-containing foods from your diet so your body is not constantly being challenged, you may even find that, once in a while, you can get away with a glass of wine at a party with no ill effects.

MANAGING FOOD INTOLERANCES

Even in simple cases of food intolerance, where there's just one problem food, it's important to read ingredient lists, ask about allergy-safe foods in restaurants, and pay attention to labels. Once, a man I know with a severe fish allergy absent-mindedly picked up a box of orange juice at the grocery store, not realizing it was fortified with fish oil, for its essential fatty acids. Fortunately, one of his children alerted him to the problem before he poured himself a glass of juice.

The more intolerances you have, the more challenging it can be to manage them. Restaurants and food manufacturers are more aware of food intolerances than they were 20 years ago, but in severe cases, people with multiple intolerances may find their only option is a rotation diet. The following passage from Allergy.org provides a good description:

> *A rotation diet is a system of controlling food allergies by eating biologically related foods on the same day and then waiting at least four days before eating them again. Such a diet can help those with food allergies in several ways.*

165

Rotation diets may help prevent the development of allergies to new foods. Any food, if eaten repetitively, can cause food allergies in allergy-prone individuals or people with "leaky guts." When my food allergies were first diagnosed, I was not told to rotate my foods. I simply eliminated the foods to which I was allergic. Four years later I had developed allergies to the foods I had used to replace the original problem foods in my diet...

A rotation diet allows you to eat foods to which you have a mild or borderline allergy and which you might not tolerate if you ate them often. Sometimes your reaction to borderline foods may depend on your stress level, other illness or infection, lack of adequate rest, or the season of the year. (For example, grain allergies tend to be more pronounced when the grass is pollinating).

A rotation diet can seem confusing, overwhelming, or confining at first. However, with a little instruction ... and practice in using a rotation diet, it will get much easier. Like hearing aids, bifocals, or any other health aid, once you get used to your rotation diet, it will become easier to use and your health will be improved by using it. *

Nowadays, you can even download an app to your smartphone to manage your rotation diet!

IT GETS BETTER

At first, diagnosing and managing food intolerances may seem like more effort than it's worth, but if you stick with it long enough to evaluate all your intolerances and develop routines to manage them, you'll likely feel so much better you'll wonder why you didn't do it sooner.

You might also find your food intolerances are helping you transition away from junk foods, taking you another step toward prevention. Perhaps you have arthritis in your family, which is an auto-immune disorder. Maybe avoiding food intolerances will strengthen your immune system, and reduce your risk of developing

---

* "How to Use a Rotation Diet," *Allergy.org,* http://www.food-allergy.org/rotation.html.

arthritis and spending the rest of your life taking palliative measures to control it.

You might even find you enjoy cooking and eating with the family more. You might notice that, as you replace your bad health habits with good ones, your children are following your example, establishing their own good health habits early in their lives. Without even meaning to, you've begun putting Generational Health First.

If you've worked through body composition and food intolerance, and your symptoms have resolved, great! Maybe stress was never part of your problem, or maybe the measure you've already taken have reduced your stress levels so much you don't need to move to the next level of the algorithm, but if you're still having symptoms, you should turn to the next chapter and read about stress evaluation.

CHAPTER 21:
TAKE CONTROL OF STRESS

A number of years ago, a woman in her thirties came into my office. She was quite overweight and very much wanted to change that, but no matter what she did, the pounds weren't coming off.

"Doctor, I am so frustrated and confused," she said. "I eat like a bird, but look at me. I've done low-carb diets, low-sugar diets, and even a gluten-free diet. I exercise regularly, too, but none of it is making any difference."

"Well, it's a good start that you're trying to lose weight and that you're exercising," I said. "It shows you're aware you have a problem and you're motivated to solve it."

She looked encouraged, so I began taking a history. She was a single parent. She'd gained weight during several years of unhappy marriage. Her self-esteem had suffered during the divorce, she said, and I wondered if she was interpreting her difficulty losing weight as proof of her inadequacies.

As we proceeded, she began sharing more details. She was under a great deal of stress: her financial situation was a constant source of worry, she often couldn't sleep, and she had a bad case of acid reflux.

Although body composition was the apparent issue, the patient's history showed that her diet, though meagre, was balanced, and she reported no symptoms that suggested food intolerance. Based on everything she'd told me, I went directly to the third level of my algorithm.

"Okay," I said, when she returned for a second visit. "The four-point salivary cortisol shows exactly what I suspected. You cortisol level is consistently high. This means your insulin level is high and you are metabolically sluggish, which explains how you can be eating so little, exercising so much, and still losing no weight."

"Oh," she said, pausing. I thought I saw relief on her face. Then she asked, "what now?"

I prescribed several remedies to bring her cortisol and insulin back to normal and we discussed ways for her to manage her stress better. Clearly, exercise alone wasn't sufficient and she couldn't afford counselling, so we focused on things she could do on her own, like making time every day for herself, stopping negative thought patterns, and visualizing the life she wanted for herself and her children.

When I saw her again six weeks later, she looked like a different person.

"Doctor, I've not only begun to lose weight, I'm actually eating a little bit more," she said. "I'm sleeping better, and I can't remember the last time I had reflux. Best of all, I feel better about myself, as if my life isn't defined by my weight or my divorce. It's like magic!"

Sometimes my patients are amazed by the difference a few small changes can make in their lives, but there is no magic in naturopathic medicine. It's all about finding the obstacles standing in the way of the body's ability to heal itself, and then taking steps to remove those obstacles.

ARE YOU LIKE THE WOMAN WHO ATE LIKE A BIRD?

If you have come this far, chances are you've already taken steps toward reducing your stress levels. Perhaps you've begun to eliminate addictive foods from your diet. Maybe you're working off cortisol with a good exercise routine. Perhaps eliminating a few foods has reduced your stress level even more. But if you're still experiencing symptoms, you may have been under stress for so long that your adrenal glands are exhausted and are no longer supplying cortisol and DHEA in a way that regulates your stress response, as I discussed in Chapter 6.

If you've been working through Dr. Jheeta's Algorithm on your own and you've come this far without the help of a naturopathic doctor, congratulations! Job well done! If all your symptoms haven't been resolved, stress may be at the root of them. Having a professional test your cortisol levels and prescribe remedies would be useful at this point. However, if that's not possible, you can still do many things to evaluate your stress levels and move forward on your own.

SIGNIFICANT SYMPTOMS OF SUSTAINED STRESS

The first step is to recognize potential signs of stress. The list of symptoms often experienced as a result of long-term stress could go on for several pages, but following are some of the most common signs:

Effects of stress on your body:

- Headache
- Muscle tension or pain
- Chest pain
- Fatigue
- Change in sex drive
- Stomach upset
- Difficulty sleeping

Effects of stress on your mood:

- Anxiety
- Restlessness
- Lack of motivation or focus
- Irritability
- Anger
- Sadness
- Depression

Effects of stress on your behaviour:

- Overeating
- Loss of appetite
- Angry outbursts
- Drug use (either prescription or illegal drugs)
- Alcohol and tobacco use
- Social withdrawal

I can't emphasize strongly enough how important it is to be proactive about recognizing these symptoms, identifying their causes, and taking steps to manage them. Stress alone, with no other apparent health issues, can trigger illness in people with any predisposition, even one they might not be aware of. That means recognizing and managing stress, without any other changes in your life or health care, could make the difference between staying healthy for years to come or developing a chronic condition such as diabetes or heart disease.

In my opinion, stress is a dramatically under-recognized, under-treated, and under-managed aspect of health. I believe making stress evaluation a central aspect of diagnosis and treatment could prevent many people from developing diseases to which they are predisposed, or at least delay the onset and prolong health for many years. According to various sources, stress plays a role in:

- **Blood Sugar Imbalance and Diabetes**: "since a principal function of cortisol is to thwart the effect of insulin – essentially rendering the cells insulin resistant – the body remains in a general insulin-resistant state when cortisol levels are chronically elevated. Over time, the pancreas struggles to keep up with the high demand for insulin, glucose levels in the blood remain high, the cells cannot get the sugar they need, and the cycle continues," says *Today's Dietician*.

- **Weight Gain and Obesity**: "repeated elevation of cortisol can lead to weight gain ... via visceral fat storage. Cortisol can mobilize triglycerides from storage and relocate them to visceral fat cells (those under the muscle, deep in the abdomen). Cortisol also aids adipocytes' development into mature fat cells." As well, "consistently high blood glucose levels along with insulin suppression lead to cells that are starved of glucose, but those cells are crying out for energy, and one way to regulate is to send hunger signals to the brain. This can lead to overeating ... another connection is cortisol's effect on appetite and cravings for high-calorie foods. Studies have demonstrated a direct association between cortisol levels and calorie intake in populations of women."

- **Immune System Suppression**: although cortisol reduces inflammation in the body, over the long term this can suppress immune function. "An unchecked immune system responding to unabated inflammation can lead to ... an increased susceptibility to colds and other illnesses, an increased risk of cancer, the tendency to develop food allergies, an increased risk of an assortment of gastrointestinal issues ... and possibly an increased risk of autoimmune disease."

- **Gastrointestinal Problems**: "in a cortisol-flooded, stressed-out body when food is consumed ... digestion and absorption are compromised, indigestion develops, and the mucosal lining becomes irritated and inflamed ... Ulcers are more common during stressful times, and many people with [IBS] and colitis report improvement in their symptoms when they master stress management."

- **Cardiovascular Disease**: "cortisol constricts blood vessels and increases blood pressure to enhance the delivery of oxygenated blood. This is advantageous for fight-or-flight situations but not perpetually. Over time, such arterial constriction and high blood pressure can lead to vessel damage and plaque buildup – the perfect scenario for a heart attack," says *Today's Dietician.* In addition, the American Heart Association notes that, "stress may affect behaviors and factors that are proven to increase heart disease risk: high blood pressure and cholesterol levels, smoking, physical inactivity, and overeating."[†]

- **Stress and Arthritis:** millions of people living with arthritis will tell you that stress makes it worse. *WebMD* tells us that "the cause may be partly chemical. When you're stressed, chemical messengers flood the brain and body; those messengers can then trigger the production of other chemicals that can cause inflammation. Regardless of the precise connection, experts tell people with RA to reduce stress in their lives."[‡]

[†] "Stress and Heart Health," American Heart Association, http://www.heart.org/HEARTORG/GettingHealthy/StressManagement/HowDoesStressAffect You/Stress-and-Heart-Health_UCM_437370_Article.jsp.
[‡] "Stress and Rheumatoid Arthritis," *WebMD,* http://www.webmd.com/rheumatoid-arthritis/ra-stress-response.

- **Stress and Cancer:** though there's no evidence that stress can cause cancer, the relationship between stress and cancer is similar to that between stress and heart disease in that coping with stress by indulging in unhealthy behaviors, such as overeating, smoking, and drinking alcohol, may increase risk of cancer indirectly. At the same time, there is evidence "that psychological stress can affect a tumor's ability to grow and spread," according to the National Cancer Institute.[δ] Also recall from Chapter 4 the way cancer can hijack blood glucose, using it to directly feed and grow its own cells, which suggests that eating a sugary diet is not good when fighting cancer.

When I say identifying and managing your stressors can be a matter of life and death, I'm not exaggerating. Researchers are always reluctant to define causal relationships (to state plainly that one thing causes another), but for your purpose of trying to understand the role of stress in your health, it's important to know that, directly or indirectly, stress can be a killer.

STRESS AND CONTROL: AN IMPORTANT RELATIONSHIP

There are some things you can't control about your stress response. For example, you may be genetically predisposed to handle stress less well than others, and that may show up in your body as depression.

In 2003, researchers found a gene that may play an important role in depression. This gene has two parts, called alleles, which can be short or long. People with two long alleles tend to have a plentiful supply of serotonin, a hormone that regulates mood. These people may be the least likely to succumb to stress by becoming depressed. People with one long and one short allele are somewhat protected from stress, but sustained stress can be a problem. People with two short alleles are often those who are most likely to become depressed due to stress. So depending somewhat on genetics, you may cope well with stress or you may not.

Even if you usually cope well with stress, your life experiences can diminish that. Perhaps you came from an abusive

---

[δ] "Psychological Stress and Cancer," *National Cancer Institute Fact Sheet,* National Institutes of Health, http://www.cancer.gov/cancertopics/factsheet/Risk/stress.

home, you've been a victim of violent crime, or you've seen active service in the military. Numerous studies have demonstrated a link between post-traumatic stress disorder (PTSD) and high blood pressure, high cholesterol levels, obesity, and heart disease.

In Chapter 6, I talked about the amount of stress a person in the role of president of the United States feels, and the greying of American presidents who spend two terms in office has been noted often. However, some studies show that people in positions of power tend to experience less stress than others. Studies have shown that they generally have lower cortisol levels than the rest of us. You might think this would be because those who cope with stress well are most likely to rise to positions of power, but other studies suggest it's just the opposite: lack of power creates stress, while being in a position of power and control relieves it.

It seems equally true that recognizing when something is beyond your control and letting go of it is an important way to manage stress. Many studies have shown that, in stressful times, people with some kind of religious faith fare better than those without it. More recent research suggests it doesn't have to be religious faith. A 2013 study showed that, during stressful times, atheists turn to science for reassurance and a sense of control – and get just as much comfort from it as people of faith do from their religious beliefs.

So, it seems that if you want to take back control of your health, you need to take back control of your stress levels. In some cases, that means reducing stressors, but even when you can't do that, you may be able to control the way you manage stress.

HOW WE ASSESS STRESS AT THE CLINIC

The first step of the stress evaluation I perform is a questionnaire, which provides a starting point for discussion. I then send the patient home with a four-point salivary cortisol test and a four-point urinary test for other adrenal hormones, as described in Chapter 14. Depending on the results, and along with information gleaned from the questionnaire and discussion, I determine a course of treatment. This could include any of the following therapies:

- **Nutritional Therapy:** even if you have a good diet, the stress response can deplete your body of essential nutrients. The results of the salivary and urinary tests should help determine whether you might benefit from supplementation with vitamins B_6 or B_{12} or minerals such as magnesium and zinc.
- **Naturopathic Therapy:** this could include a wide variety of vitamins (such as B complex), herbal treatments (such as Asian ginseng or ashwagandha, an Ayurvedic medicine), homeopathic remedies, and Traditional Chinese Medicines (TCM), sometimes delivered intravenously.
- **Allopathic Therapy:** in many jurisdictions, ND/NMDs can now prescribe pharmaceuticals. I always consider preventive treatments first, but sometimes a palliative treatment is more appropriate. For example, if a woman is stressed because her partner is terminally ill, her teenager is acting out, and she's lost her job after taking too many personal days, suggesting she learn better stress management techniques is unlikely to help. There are situations in which we should all be grateful for pharmaceutical interventions, and I will gladly either refer her to an MD, or work with an MD to prescribe appropriate drugs when it's clear little else will help.
- **Cognitive Behavioural Therapy**[δ]**:** I use this term broadly to describe any set of therapeutic counselling and behaviour modification techniques that can be combined effectively with other nutritional, naturopathic, and allopathic therapies to help the patient change thoughts and behaviours, and address physical issues, to manage stress better.

[δ] "CBT is a psychological treatment that addresses the interactions between how we think, feel and behave. It is usually time-limited (approximately 10–20 sessions), focuses on current problems and follows a structured style of intervention. . . . CBT is less like a single intervention and more like a family of treatments and practices. Practitioners of CBT may emphasize different aspects of treatment (cognitive, emotional, or behavioural) based on the training of the practitioner. . . . What gets used (that is, which technique for which problem) is what has been proven effective and the techniques themselves derive from science (for example, the 'behavioural experiments' used to help people overcome feared objects or situations). CBT has been studied and effectively implemented with persons who have multiple and complex needs, and who may be receiving additional forms of treatment, or have had no success with other kinds of treatment." From http://www.health.gov.bc.ca/library/publications/year/2007/MHA_CognitiveBehaviouralThe rapy.pdf.

About six to eight weeks after the initial salivary and urinary tests, I perform them a second time to determine whether cortisol levels, and other markers of adrenal function, have returned to normal.

HOW YOU CAN ASSESS YOUR STRESS AT HOME

Perhaps the most important result of doing the questionnaire is that it can raise a patient's awareness of the stress he's living with. I'm often amazed when patients tell me what they're coping with daily. In our culture, we're taught that strength means, "stay calm and carry on." We're told talking about our problems is whining, but there's a difference between whining and seeking support for the challenges you face.

If I ask most people (not patients) what's causing their stress, they're likely to say, "Oh, it's not that bad," and change the subject. It's only when patients have to answer direct questions that they start thinking, talking, and writing about the stress they're managing. Coping with stress is like any other problem. You have to know what the problem is before you can deal with it.

Here are some questions I ask patients to get them thinking and talking about the stressors in their lives. If you're ready to start dealing with stress in your life, grab a pen and paper, get comfortable, and start writing. If you're like many people, you'll find once you start, the answers will begin flowing – and you might be surprised what you learn about yourself:

- How are you sleeping? More or less than usual? Are you going to bed and rising around the same time every day? Are you waking up rested, or still tired?
- What physical aches and pains are you feeling? Even if you think they're the result of an exercise injury or sitting at your desk, make note of them.
- Is anything upsetting you emotionally? Problems at work? Struggles with financial issues? Tension in your relationships with you partner, your children, or your extended family?

176

- Have you been thinking about childhood events recently? Do you have feelings about things you think could or should have gone differently?
- What, if any, drugs are you taking? Prescription medications? Recreational drugs or alcohol? How often do you use them? Do you most often use them socially, or when you feel stressed?
- Have there been any changes in your appetite lately? Are you eating more or less? Are there any particular foods you've been craving?
- Has your weight been fluctuating? Has it gone up or down in direct relationship with the amount you've been eating? Or do you seem to be gaining or losing weight for no reason?
- How has your mood been? Have you felt like your emotional energy is good? Or have you been feeling a bit down? Have you had difficulty with concentration, focus, or memory?
- What about your physical energy? Have you felt motivated and driven to do things? Or have you felt like you just don't have the energy to do the things you'd like to do?
- What sort of exercise have you been getting? Have you been dragging yourself out for a small bit of exercise and saying that's enough? Or feeling like no amount of high-intensity exercise is enough?

Once you've completed the questionnaire, review your responses and organize them from worst to least. Then put them in a different order, from those you have least control over to those you have most control over. Are there any patterns? You might begin to see, as research has shown, that the things you find most stressful are the things you can control the least.

PRIORITIZE AND ORGANIZE

Just because some things in your life are beyond your control doesn't mean there's nothing you can do about your stress. First, you can look at what you can control and decide how to deal with that. Then, you can look at what you can't control and decide how to stop stressing about things you can't change anyways.

One way to think about stress is to look at your daily life, list the things you consider most important to accomplish each day, and organize your day around them. Let's say this book is stressing you out because it's telling you to eat a good breakfast with your kids every day but you can't imagine how you would do that and still get them to school on time and yourself to work on time. You'd have to get up earlier, but you already struggle to sleep at night, often sleeping through your alarm, and then let the kids eat a sugary cereal even though you know the health risks of eating processed foods.

Maybe there's a different way to look at it. Maybe, you could make breakfast a priority and change other things to accommodate it. Maybe if you have a hard time sleeping, it's because you're still wound up from your day. Maybe you could stop watching TV 60 minutes earlier, and use that time to make the next day's lunches to take time demands off the morning, and to have your shower at night to help you unwind. Then you could go to bed at the same time, but maybe get to sleep better. You could get up at the same time, and have enough time for a good breakfast with the kids.

If what researchers say about breakfast is right, you could not only reduce your stress, but also take control of your body composition issues. You could move toward prevention and away from palliation by possibly reducing your risk of any chronic diseases related to body composition and stress, which should be under better control just by having a good breakfast with the family. You could replace your own bad health habits with good ones, and teach good health habits to your children – all because you decided to take control of one thing that was causing you stress.

REDUCE STRESS WITH ROUTINES

Do you know that one of the most stressful things we do in a day is make decisions? How many times in a day do you make decisions? Is it necessary for you to make all those decisions each day? Or are there some things you could just make part of your routine to take decision-making stress out of your day? Try these ideas on for size:

- Some people find that deciding on a "uniform" to wear every day – whether it's a blue suit and tie or jeans and a white t-shirt – takes one decision-making element out of their day and reduces stress.

178

- A friend of mine makes a meal plan for the coming week every Saturday. It simplifies grocery shopping and cooking because it concentrates the decision-making into five minutes once a week.
- What about creating a daily plan? List the things you'd most like to accomplish each day and then set a time for each of them. (Read a novel: 1 hour. Exercise: 45 minutes.) When the allotted time is up, move on to the next thing, knowing you'll have the same opportunity the next day.

UTILIZE THE POWER OF VISUALIZATION

If you're like most people, you spend a lot of time worrying about what will happen if your dreams don't come true. Some people believe we attract whatever we spend the most time thinking about. So thinking about positive things can affect our lives positively, and thinking about negative things can have the opposite effect.

You don't have to be a master of visualization to put its power to work for you. For now, start with a simple idea: Visualize an image of you and your family doing something you enjoy together. Maybe it's riding your bikes in the sun or playing a board game on a rainy day. Imagine the colours, sounds, and smells. Enjoy the way you feel when you think about it.

Now visualize you and your family a few years from now. Your children are older and your activities have changed, but you're still spending time together, healthy and happy. Again, imagine the sights, sounds, colours, and the way you feel.

Keep changing the visualization until you see yourself living a long, happy, healthy life together with your family. See the benefits you'll enjoy by being healthier than you are now. The healthier you are, the more energy you'll have to do the things you want with your family, and for yourself. The healthier your body and mind become, the more vibrant your physical appearance will be, and the more positive your outlook on life – all because you started visualizing what you wanted.

DO WHAT WORKS FOR YOU

Even if you don't believe in visualization, you can look for upsides in whatever happens. I'm not talking about denying your stressors; that won't make them go away. I'm talking about considering the things that happen to you from all angles, and choosing how you're going to look at them. Are you going to let yourself feel burdened over things that have already happened? Or are you going to say, "It's done. What can I do now to make the best of it?"

Thinking about your stressors also allows you to put them into categories of what you can and can't control. Taking charge of things you can control can often help you let go of things you can't. I live on Canada's west coast, in an earthquake zone. Every so often, there's a tremor and the media warn us about the "big one" coming sometime in the next century. I could let myself worry about that, but it wouldn't do any good because I can't control it. What I can control is whether I'm prepared for it. If I have an earthquake kit and I keep it up to date, I know I've done everything I can, and I can let go of the rest because it's beyond my control anyway.

How many things are there in your life that you might stress about less if you were to figure out what parts you can control, do what you can, and let go of the rest? Will you make the effort to do that now that you know not doing so might be harming your health?

GETTING THROUGH CHANGE

There's an adage that it takes 21 days to form a new routine. As it turns out, this is false; it actually takes about two months. Maybe that's why some people have a hard time making changes. They expect it should become habit more quickly than is realistic. Maybe if you go into changing habits with that knowledge, it will help you keep track of the days until what seems like an impossible task simply becomes a new habit.

Sixty days still seems like a pretty long time. There are some things I don't know if I could keep up for that long.

Okay. But what if, instead of focusing on how hard it might be to change your routines, you try to focus on the bigger picture? What if you compare 60 days of effort to change a bad health habit into a good one, and set a good example for your children, with the possible lifelong consequences of not changing?

But even if I make the effort, there's no guarantee. I could still get ill with something hereditary, and then my effort wouldn't make any difference.

There are no guarantees. But even if you did still get sick, would you really say your effort didn't make any difference? If you were able to overcome your stress and feel healthier, wouldn't that make a difference? If you were able to make better use of your time with your family, wouldn't that make a difference? If you were able to teach your children to trade bad health habits for good ones, wouldn't that make a difference? When you look at the big picture of health, does 60 days out of your whole life still seem like such a big deal? Or does the importance of making the change seem a little bigger?

STILL EXPERIENCING SYMPTOMS OF STRESS?

If you've worked your way through your stressors as much as you can and you're still having difficulties, you may have reached the limit of what you can do to improve your chronic health issues on our own. Like the woman in the story at the beginning of this chapter, you may need the help of an ND/NMD to assess your stress and help you make necessary changes.

Although there are websites where you can order your own four-point salivary cortisol test and send it off to a laboratory for appraisal, I don't recommend this approach. If you're going to spend what that will cost, you're better off consulting with an ND/NMD who can not only perform the assessment, but recommend specific supplements to normalize your cortisol levels. I'll cover what to look for in a qualified ND/NMD in the next chapter.

CHAPTER 22:
TAKE CONTROL OF TOXIC LOAD

The word "dementia" evokes fear in most people's minds. It's a slowly progressing disease with devastating consequences. Most often when patients receive this diagnosis, they are told there appears to be no known cause and no real treatment options exist.

Some years ago, I had such a patient. At 76 years old, he was quite healthy. He'd begun to notice he was becoming forgetful, which he ignored, as most of us would. However, when he began to forget names and faces, even of old friends and relatives, he took notice.

Then he started becoming delusional about activities and tasks he claimed to have done or needed to do, such as shopping. He missed appointments. These symptoms are often signs of major neurological issues. His allopathic doctor referred him to a specialist, who made the bleak diagnoses of dementia. Progression, his doctor told him, was inevitable.

He came to my office seeking someone who could offer him some hope. On taking his history, I found nothing remarkable. Yet he seemed so healthy overall that it was hard to believe that this was "it" for him. The only possible reprieve I could think of was toxic exposure. He couldn't remember anything that might have caused it, but on a hunch I asked his permission to perform a urinalysis for toxic heavy metals, and he agreed.

"I have bad news, and I have good news," I said when he returned to my office.

"Okay," he said, "let's hear the bad news."

"There are high levels of mercury, lead, and thallium in your urine," I said.

"That doesn't sound good," he said. "What's the good news?"

"This could explain why you're having dementia-like symptoms," I said.

"Dementia-like," he said. "You mean, not dementia?"

"I can't make any promises," I said. "But we can proceed with a detoxification protocol for a few months and see what happens."

"Whatever happens," he said, "it can't be worse than what the other doctors have prepared me for."

In addition to detoxification therapy, I recommended several nutraceutical supplements appropriate to enhancing neurological function in a man of his age. I also suggested he try several cognitive enhancement exercises available online.

He complied with all my recommendations, his rate of cognitive degeneration stabilized, and his memory improved. According to his own assessment, he was doing better.

I am uncertain how things worked out for this man and I have not seen him again; there was no more I could have done for him in any case, but I include this story to highlight the fact that toxic exposure can affect people in ways we don't think of and also because this man walked into my office with no hope, and left feeling some degree of empowerment instead of only despair. He regained hope in a situation that felt hopeless. To him, that meant something.

SHIFTING THE BALANCE OF CONTROL

You might think that when striving to provide you with empowering information on toxic load, I would suggest you do a "cleanse." You could find at least a dozen "cleansing" products in stores and dozens more online. I have no doubt almost any of them would help you feel better.

But then, you would likely also feel better if you were to stop eating processed foods and eating to excess, and start eating three healthy meals each day, beginning with breakfast and ensuring that each meal includes, if possible, pesticide-free and medication-free foods. You would feel even better if you were to drink lots of water, exercise daily, and get enough sleep every night.

If you find that the structure provided by a particular cleansing program helps you stay on track with your efforts to take control of your health, then by all means, do what works. But beyond that, there's no evidence that any commercial product or diet will be more effective than simply following some of the common sense steps I've covered in this book.

However, if you've worked through all the steps in this book and you're still experiencing symptoms, it's unlikely any product you buy in a store or online is going to provide more than transient help. If this is the case for you, you need to find someone who is qualified, have toxins in your blood checked through a laboratory, and follow recommended detoxification protocols under professional guidance.

This does not mean you are not still in control of your health but that the balance of control is shifting. Your empowerment now comes through understanding what's happening with your health and finding a qualified professional to help you deal with it. I can provide two types of empowerment here. First, I can offer more information on some of the most common toxins in daily life with suggestions for reducing their levels in your food and environment. Second, I can offer guidance as to how to find a naturopathic doctor, and what to look for to be sure you are finding a qualified professional.

MINIMIZE EVERYDAY TOXIC EXPOSURE

Dr. Joseph Mercola, who runs the second most-visited health website in the world (after *WebMD*) and the first most-visited integrated health website, tells us a great deal about everyday exposure to toxins. For example, he describes several studies connecting traffic pollution with increased risk of heart disease. A German study notes a link between atherosclerosis and long-term exposure to particulate matter from living close to major roadways. French researchers linked four out of five major traffic pollutants (carbon monoxide, nitrogen dioxide, sulphur dioxide, and particulate matter) with increased risk of heart attack. An American study showed greater risk of atherosclerosis among those who lived in more polluted areas than those in less polluted areas.

That's good to know, but it's not always practical to just pick up and move. Are there other ways to reduce toxic exposure?

One thing to pay attention to, says Mercola, is personal care products and cosmetics. In 2013, *Scientific American* reported that a chemical called *cyclic siloxanes*, which is used in personal care products such as deodorants, lotions, and conditioners, is present at alarming levels in the air in the city of Chicago, and probably other cities. A study in *Environmental Health Perspectives* confirms previous findings of nine heavy metals, including lead, cadmium, chromium, and aluminum, in 32 lipsticks and lip glosses, and cautions that children should not play with these cosmetics

That sounds like a high price for beauty.

Not only personal beauty, but also home beauty. Mercola goes on to say home products have become such significant sources of toxicity, too. In 2013, nearly four dozen health and environmental groups banded together to launch a campaign against big-box retailers including Kroger, Walgreens, Home Depot, CVS Caremark, Lowe's, Best Buy, and Safeway over the use of more than 100 toxic chemicals in products ranging from vinyl flooring to wrinkle-free and stain-resistant fabrics and even food packaging.

It seems almost inescapable. How do these toxic chemicals affect us?

They've been linked with cancer, infertility, learning disabilities, and behavioural problems, among other things. It's especially concerning when you consider Mercola's statement that "a typical American comes in regular contact with some 6,000 chemicals and an untold number of potentially toxic substances on a less frequent basis, [many of which] have never been fully tested for safety."[†]

Okay, but other than moving away from traffic and completely renovating our homes, what can we do to minimize exposure?

Mercola has the following recommendations, and you'll find more in Chapter 25, where I discuss taking back control of your children's health:

1. As much as possible, buy and eat organic produce and free-range, organic foods.
2. Rather than eating conventional or farm-raised fish, supplement with a high-quality purified krill oil, or eat wild fish.

[†] "Top Three Sources of Toxic Exposures: Traffic, Personal Care and Plastic Products," Dr. Joseph Mercola, *Mercola.com,* May 15, 2013, http://articles.mercola.com/sites/articles/archive/2013/05/15/toxic-chemical-exposure.aspx#_edn2.

3. Eat mostly raw, fresh foods, steering clear of processed, prepackaged foods of all kinds.
4. Store your food and beverages in glass rather than plastic, and avoid using plastic wrap and canned foods.
5. Have your tap water tested and, if contaminants are found, install an appropriate water filter.
6. Only use natural cleaning products in your home.
7. Switch over to natural brands of toiletries such as shampoo, toothpaste, antiperspirants, and cosmetics.
8. Avoid using artificial air fresheners, dryer sheets, fabric softeners, or other synthetic fragrances.
9. Replace your Teflon pots and pans with ceramic or glass cookware or a safe nonstick pan.
10. When redoing your home, look for toxin-free alternatives to regular paint and vinyl floor coverings.
11. Replace your vinyl shower curtain with a fabric one or install a glass shower door.
12. Limit your use of drugs (over-the-counter and prescriptions) as much as possible.
13. Avoid spraying pesticides around your home or insect repellants that contain DEET on your body. There are safe, effective, and natural alternatives out there.

Most naturopathic doctors will perform some form of toxic evaluation. Blood serum levels of toxins, urinary excretion of toxins, and/or bioenergetics toxic evaluation. Once a toxic load evaluation is complete, treatment options can vary dramatically.

Chelation is a method commonly used to assist the body's ability to bind and eliminate heavy metals through the urine. Treatments can be done using oral supplements or Intravenous therapy. Other methods include the use of nutraceuticals to assist in the body's own detoxification pathway through the liver and lymphatic system. Another useful option is the use of powerful nutrients such as bioflavonoids, carotenoids, and antioxidants to protect against the damaging effects of toxins. Here is a list of some promising and exciting detoxification nutrients:

- Intravenous Glutathione peroxidase therapy

- Cilantro
- Blue green algae
- Quercitin
- Turmeric
- Milk thistle
- Andrographis
- Selenium
- Zinc

FINDING A NATUROPATHIC MEDICAL DOCTOR

The next most empowering advice I can offer is how to find a qualified naturopathic doctor to work with. This is not as simple as finding an allopathic doctor. Allopathic medicine is such a large and well-regulated profession that it's highly unlikely you'll ever find an allopathic doctor who was not educated at an accredited institution and licensed to practice in your area.

Naturopathy is a much younger and smaller profession. It is unfortunately still possible to find men and women who say they practice naturopathic medicine but who have not been trained at an accredited institution. Accreditation and licensing exist to protect patients by screening out those who have not been trained to standards agreed upon by those professionals who have received the arduous training that our profession requires.

To be qualified, an individual must have been educated at an accredited institution and practice under the designation Naturopathic Doctor (ND) or Naturopathic Medical Doctor (NMD). I strongly advise you not to spend your time or money on a person who simply calls himself a "naturopath." If he is not using the designation ND or NMD, he has likely not been trained at an accredited naturopathic college or university. Stay away!

The best way to find a properly trained ND or NMD is to visit the websites of the Canadian Association of Naturopathic Doctors (www.cand.ca) or the American Association of Naturopathic Physicians (naturopathic.org). If you are in any doubt about the qualifications of the professional you are considering, check her credentials against the following complete list of accredited naturopathic colleges and universities in Canada and the US:

- Bastyr University, Washington
- Bastyr University, California Campus
- National College of Natural Medicine, Oregon
- National University of Health Sciences, Illinois
- Southwest College of Naturopathic Medicine, Arizona
- University of Bridgeport College of Naturopathic Medicine, Connecticut
- Canadian College of Naturopathic Medicine, Ontario, Canada
- Boucher Institute of Naturopathic Medicine, British Columbia, Canada

If you do not find the degree-granting institution where your ND or NMD says he was educated, ask him for the name and location of the school from which he graduated and contact the national association in your country to determine if they recognize it as providing education up to their standards. It may be an accredited school in another country. However, it could also be one of many unaccredited schools that unfortunately continue to undermine the credibility of our profession.

In the US, NDs and NMDs are licensed to practice in Alaska, Arizona, California, Colorado, Connecticut, District of Columbia, Hawaii, Kansas, Maine, Maryland, Minnesota, Montana, New Hampshire, North Dakota, Oregon, Utah, Vermont, and Washington, as well as Puerto Rico and the Virgin Islands. In Canada, there are licensing bodies in Alberta, British Columbia, Manitoba, Ontario, and Saskatchewan, and professional associations in all provinces and territories except Nunavut.

If you live in a state or province that does not regulate the profession through a licensing body, you must be particularly diligent in checking that the professional you are considering has graduated with an appropriate degree from one of the colleges or universities I've listed. There is no more empowering advice I can provide at this point than to be certain that the professional you're seeing is fully qualified to be entrusted with your health.

WHAT DO ND/NMDS STUDY?

I'm often asked how an ND/NMD's education compares with that of an MD. As for any medical school, an applicant to an accredited naturopathic college requires a four-year Bachelor of Science degree from a recognized university, including standard pre-medical courses. (Some naturopathic schools provide courses to allow those with another degree to upgrade their understanding of pre-medical science prior to beginning the program. This is also true for allopathic medical students.)

Like medical doctors, naturopathic physicians then complete a four-year graduate-level program. For NDs and NMDs, this includes basic sciences, naturopathic therapies and techniques, diagnostic techniques and tests, specialty courses, clinical sciences, and clinical training. Graduates receive a degree of ND or NMD, depending on where the degree is issued. Although postdoctoral (residency) training is not required, some graduates pursue residency opportunities.

WHAT TO EXPECT ON YOUR FIRST VISIT

Your first visit with an ND or NMD may come as a surprise. An initial visit may last an hour or more, as the ND or NMD will take your health history, ask about your diet, stress levels, and use of tobacco and alcohol, and discuss why you're there. He may perform an examination and order diagnostic tests, set up an individual strategy for managing your health issues, and if necessary refer you to another health care practitioner.

Follow-up visits are likely to be less lengthy, but you may still be surprised by the amount of time an ND or NMD will spend with you. The goal of naturopathic medicine is not to diagnose disease and provide palliative care, but to understand your symptoms and prevent them from developing into disease. This takes time, so time is built into the appointment structure. Make the most of it. Don't go to your appointment expecting to be in and out quickly. Plan around the time your ND or NMD will spend with you. Be sure to consider yourself as much of a priority as your naturopathic doctor considers you.

CHAPTER 23:
TAKE CONTROL OF AGING

Some time ago, I treated a 56-year-old woman for a combination of concerns, including anxiety, insomnia, poor libido, and dyspareunia (painful intercourse). She worked part time as an administrator.

"I don't think my anxiety is psychological," she said. "I don't feel particularly stressed. Other than the part-time work, I'm retired."

"Okay," I said, thinking I should take a different approach. "When did menopause begin for you?"

"When I was 37," she said.

That told me the root cause of her problems was likely premature aging.

Her allopathic doctor had prescribed a drug called estrogel, a topical gel applied daily to increase the body's levels of estradiol and lessen symptoms of menopause. She was also taking lorazepam, though she was perplexed as to why this had been prescribed.

"My husband and I are financially stable," she said. "I have no emotional issues. Why would my doctor give me an anti-anxiety medication? I'm so frustrated by having no sex life, and the lorazepam seems to be making matters worse. I'm also concerned about long-term effects of estrogen replacement. Isn't it connected with cancer?"

"Yes," I said, "it is. And you are not wrong about lorazepam. Decreased libido can be an adverse effect. "

Age management testing revealed low testosterone, low estrogen, low IGF1, and high SHBG. As you may recall from Chapter 9, SHBG (sex hormone binding globulin) regulates estrogen and testosterone, so this explained why her testosterone and estrogen levels were low. SHBG naturally diminishes with age, contributing to everything from wrinkled skin to osteoarthritis, but this patient was well ahead of a normal aging schedule. IGF-1 (insulin-like growth factor) is important in preventing cellular breakdown, and a low level is a clear indicator of accelerated aging.

I immediately started her on a protocol of antioxidant vitamins and botanical supplements to bring these parameters closer to normal for her chronological age. The results were quick and outstanding. Stabilizing her estrogen levels eliminated her anxiety and sleep issues, and she was able to withdraw from the lorazepam and the estradiol. Raising her free testosterone had a quick and positive impact on her libido. Slowly her dyspareunia improved, also.

Although I had not set out to address any other issues, the protocol also helped bring her body composition closer to what she wanted, and reduced her homocysteine levels, which in turn reduces risk of heart disease. The last time I saw her, she was a different woman than the one I'd first met, happy and confident. Even as we age, it's amazing what normal hormone levels and a little sexual activity will do for our sense of well-being.

MANAGE WELLNESS AND AGING

If you have worked through the first four stages of Dr. Jheeta's Algorithm and you are still having symptoms, it's time to move to the next stage. As explained in Chapter 8, the next stage will depend on whether you are under or over 40. If you are under 40 and still have symptoms, wellness evaluation and treatment are unlikely to address your concerns. If you were a patient at the clinic, I would suggest Specialized Health Care, which could include a combination of naturopathic and allopathic treatments.

As mentioned earlier, NDs in many jurisdictions are now licensed to prescribe an extensive list of drugs, such as antibiotics, anticonvulsants, and antidepressants. Because NDs also understand the therapeutic uses and interactions of a wide variety of nutraceuticals (vitamins, minerals, and other nutritional supplements and botanical remedies), they are well equipped to use allopathic drugs and naturopathic remedies in combination.

If you are over 40, I would proceed to the final stage of the algorithm, the Wellness or Age Management Evaluation. I sometimes see patients who are 40 years old but whose bodies have the characteristics of a 50-year-old. Many factors can influence premature aging, but some of the most common factors include:

- Genetic predisposition
- Poor dietary habits
- Lack of exercise
- Weight gain
- Physical or emotional trauma
- Use of alcohol, tobacco, or caffeine
- Use of OTC or prescription drugs
- Recreational use of either prescription or "street" drugs
- Exposure to environmental toxins
- Exposure to toxins in foods

This is not simply a matter of looking older than we are. It has more to do with the levels of various hormones and proteins in our bodies (I provided a list in Chapter 8), which act as markers of age and predictors of disease. These markers influence things like how well our bodies respond to environmental toxins, fend off illness, or recover from injury. If the levels of these markers are too high, too low, or unstable, it can predict greater risk for developing chronic degenerative diseases than would be normal for our age.

I evaluate the levels of these markers in a patient's body through a blood sample, and then recommend treatments to help normalize these levels. Treatments could include nutritional or botanical supplements, Ayurvedic medicines, Traditional Chinese Medicines, or anything else experience has proven useful.

WHY SUPPLEMENT?

Patients often ask me, "Do I need to take supplements?" The answer is complicated. I don't believe taking massive amounts of random supplements is a wise practice for a number of reasons. First, the average person is not in a position to know what supplements might serve their needs best, and taking every supplement on the store shelf without consulting a professional is kind of like buying up every OTC drug and taking it without knowing why. It doesn't make sense.

Second, many supplements have adverse effects, just like drugs. For example, random high doses of vitamin C to ward off cold and flu can cause gas, bloating, or diarrhea. Vitamin B supplements are difficult for some people to digest and can cause or exacerbate reflux. You also can't assume that just because a supplement is natural, it's safe. Some supplements are not even available in some countries because they have the potential to put people in the hospital.

Third, supplements come in different forms and some are more effective than others. You've probably heard people say taking supplements just gives you expensive urine. If you buy cheap supplements without knowing which forms of each nutrient work best for which purposes, how to evaluate the ingredients on the label, or what the threshold is for your body to absorb that supplement, you probably will end up with expensive urine.

It's a different story if you are seeing a qualified professional who recommends supplements to meet your needs. Most patients have specific requirements, for example, the patients that take some form of prescription medication. Among the adverse effects of most prescription drugs is that they can deplete important nutrients – in fact, much of the time, the adverse effects are linked to these depletions – and a naturopathic doctor may recommend supplements to compensate. For other patients, lifestyle habits such as alcohol and cigarette use have led to nutrient depletion. Again, a naturopathic doctor knows which nutrients are most likely to have been depleted and can recommend appropriate supplements.

Children, youth, and young adults who have grown up eating nutritionally void foods can suffer health issues as a result. Their deficiencies generally do not reach the level required in allopathic medicine to declare a disease of deficiency (such as rickets, caused by low vitamin D, or scurvy by low vitamin C), but it only makes sense that there is a level of nutritional status that falls between a level required for optimal health and a level so low as to cause a disease of severe deficiency. In fact, researchers have defined many symptoms of low to moderate deficiencies. I have found supplements very effective in young people who have grown up eating nutrient-deprived junk-food diets.

These are not the only reasons to supplement, but a few examples. As mentioned in Chapter 2, research on the decreased nutritional value of mass produced foods is still controversial, but my opinion is that we can no longer depend on a healthy diet to supply all the nutrition we need. In our increasingly toxic world, our bodies need vital nutrients to combat the impacts of environmental toxicity, because I'm convinced the quality of our food is diminishing. I believe the time will come when research will support this and, at that time, those who have taken precautions will be glad they did.

SEVEN SUPER SUPPLEMENTS

Once I have evaluated a patient's markers of aging, their total health picture will tell me what supplements they need. If you have been through the full evaluation process with a naturopathic doctor, they may already have recommended certain supplements. If you have worked through the first few levels of the algorithm on your own, you may be reasonably satisfied with the results but wonder if there's anything else you might do to manage wellness and aging. The following is a list of what I consider the seven most important supplements for the average person as they move into middle age. I recommend these with the goal of preventing chronic disease, and avoiding the palliative care options too many patients are left with as a result of choosing not to take preventive measures before it was too late:

- Vitamin D

  According to research done at the University of Calgary, 97% of Canadians are deficient in vitamin D at some point in the year, most commonly between October and April when the days grow short for the sun to provide enough vitamin D. Vitamin D promotes absorption of calcium, which is essential for normal bone growth and therefore helps prevent osteoporosis.

  Hundreds of studies now link vitamin D deficiency with higher rates of Alzheimer's disease and other forms of cognitive impairment in the elderly, as well as congestive heart failure and coronary heart disease. Adequate vitamin D may improve insulin sensitivity in those with Type I diabetes, and reduce risk of developing Type II diabetes in later life.

Vitamin D is a relatively new area of research interest, but it is proving to be a far more important nutrient than previously suspected. Researchers are currently assessing whether recommendations for daily vitamin D intake need to be revised. As we age, and particularly if we live where the days grow short for several months of the year, we can't go wrong with vitamin D supplements.

- Coenzyme Q10

  I believe the importance of this nutrient is under rated. CoQ10 is found in every cell in the body and research has demonstrated its role in preventing heart failure. The fact that heart failure is the number one killer in North America earns CoQ10 its place among the Seven Super Supplements.

  "Many medical studies demonstrate supplemental CoQ10's beneficial effects, most of which stem from its vital role in oxygen utilization and energy production, particularly in heart muscle cells," writes Dr. Andrew Weil. CoQ10 "assists in maintaining the normal oxidative state of LDL cholesterol, helps assure circulatory health, and supports optimal functioning of the heart muscle."[*] There is also evidence that people taking statin drugs are at risk of CoQ10 deficiency.

  CoQ10 has also been studied for its role in the treatment of Parkinson's disease. Preliminary research has shown a correlation between low CoQ10 levels and Parkinson's. A correlation is not a causal relationship; correlation means two things often happen together, whereas causation means the deficiency causes the problem and perhaps implies supplementation could alleviate it. However, although causation has not been proven, the Mayo Clinic notes "there is promising evidence in support of the use of CoQ10 for this condition."[†]

---

[*] "Coenzyme Q10," by Dr. Andrew Weil, *Weil*,
http://www.drweil.com/drw/u/ART03367/Coenzyme-Q10-CoQ10.html.
[†] "Coenzyme Q10 Evidence," Mayo Clinic, http://www.mayoclinic.org/drugs-supplements/coenzyme-q10/evidence/hrb-20059019.

- Magnesium

Magnesium, the fourth most-abundant mineral in the body, is best known for its roles in heart health, bone density, muscle function, diabetes, and hypertension. "Magnesium is essential to heart health," according to the University of Maryland Medical Centre. "Magnesium and calcium work together at very precise ratios to ensure your heart functions properly." [‡]

Magnesium is also an important trace mineral in bone matrix, and some consider it as essential in preventing and treating osteoporosis as calcium and vitamin D. Muscle spasms, cramps, and restless legs syndrome have all been linked with magnesium deficiency.

"Magnesium plays a central role in the secretion and action of insulin. Without adequate magnesium levels within the body's cells, control over blood-sugar level is impossible." Finally, in areas where there is plenty of magnesium in the natural water supply, fewer people suffer from high blood pressure.

- Selenium

Selenium is an essential trace mineral and antioxidant that is naturally present in the soil and water. Research shows that where selenium is naturally low, rates of certain conditions are higher. These conditions include cancer, heart disease, inflammatory diseases, and premature aging.

Selenium has proven effective in fighting some types of cancer, though it seems most strongly related with lower rates of prostate cancer. Selenium is also associated with lower rates of death among those with cancer. Selenium is vital in making and using glutathione peroxidase. This powerful antioxidant plays an important role in immune function, which reduces the risk of developing cancer and many chronic degenerative illnesses associated with aging.

However, selenium supplements are only effective if you have a deficiency. You may be low in selenium if you "smoke cigarettes, drink alcohol, take birth control pills, or have a condition that

[‡] "Magnesium Overview," University of Maryland Medical Center, http://umm.edu/health/medical/altmed/supplement/magnesium.

prevents your body from absorbing enough selenium such as Crohn's disease or ulcerative colitis."[δ]

- Folic Acid

  Folic acid is the most common nutrient deficiency in the world. As it is most plentiful in green leafy vegetables, deficiency is often a product of a diet too focused on animal protein. As with all the other B vitamins, folic acid deficiency is often associated with alcoholism.

  Folic acid deficiency affects all cells of the body because it is needed to produce new cells. Inadequate folic acid in the first weeks after conception can lead to birth defects such as spina bifida, but folic acid remains important throughout life, particularly for brain function. Folic acid and B_{12} are often low in patients with depression. Taking folic acid can have a mild impact on depression; taken with antidepressants, it may boost the drugs' effectiveness.

  Folic acid also seems to provide some protection against heart disease and stroke. Adequate levels of B_6, B_{12}, and folic acid appear to lower homocysteine levels. As high homocysteine levels are linked with increased risk of heart disease and stroke, lowering them should reduce this risk.

- Zinc

  "Adequate zinc levels are essential to good health," writes Michael T. Murray, a well-known ND. "The benefits of zinc are extensive because it is involved in so many enzyme and body functions. By necessity, the discussion ... focuses on zinc's effects on immune function, wound healing, sensory functions, sexual function, and skin health."[φ]

[δ] "Selenium Overview," University of Maryland Medical Center, http://umm.edu/health/medical/altmed/supplement/selenium.
[φ] *The Encyclopedia of Nutritional Supplements,* Michael T. Murray, ND, Rocklin, CA: Prima Publishing, 1996. Learn more about Dr. Murray at http://doctormurray.com/.

Zinc supplements are most commonly recommended to improve immune function and wound healing, which naturally become depressed with age; zinc intake in older adults may be low. Zinc levels may also be low in people with Crohn's disease, colitis, and other intestinal issues, as well as vegetarians, pregnant and lactating women, and alcoholics.

Studies have shown zinc supplements effective in reducing length and severity of infections ranging from colds to pneumonia, particularly in the elderly; in reducing diarrhea in children in developing countries; in supporting wound healing, particularly in the elderly; and in combination with other minerals in slowing the progression of age-related macular degeneration.

- Vitamin C

  Vitamin C has three main roles in the body: it's crucial in the manufacture of collagen, a protein in the tissues that literally holds our bodies together; it's the warrior of the immune system, playing several vital roles in fighting disease; and it's a powerful antioxidant, critical to staving off the ravages of many chronic degenerative diseases.

  According to *WebMD*, "vitamin C is one of the safest and most effective nutrients ... It may not be the cure for the common cold (though it's thought to help prevent more serious complications). But the benefits of vitamin C may include protection against immune system deficiencies, cardiovascular disease, prenatal health problems, eye disease, and even skin wrinkling.

  A recent study published in *Seminars in Preventive and Alternative Medicine* that looked at over 100 studies over 10 years revealed a growing list of benefits of vitamin C.

  'Higher blood levels of vitamin C may be the ideal nutrition marker for overall health,' says [a researcher at] the University of Michigan. 'The more we study vitamin C, the better our understanding of how diverse it is in protecting our health, from cardiovascular disease, cancer, stroke, eye health [and] immunity to living longer.'"[β]

RECHARGE YOUR BATTERIES WITH SLEEP AND WATER

There are two other important factors in wellness that I haven't discussed in the context of the algorithm. While both have healing properties, I can't prescribe them in the same way I would prescribe supplements or therapies. I can only advise you to get plenty of both. Those factors are sleep and water.

If you have a busy, stressful life, you need plenty of energy to cope with it. Some of that energy comes from food, but a lot of it comes from sleep. There is a direct two-way relationship between sleep and health: the more sleep you get, the healthier you tend to be, and the healthier you are, the better you tend to sleep.

Sleep may be the most neglected factor in health. In these busy times, when we need arguably more sleep to cope with the pressures of living, we're getting less. According to a 2002 study by the National Sleep Foundation, "before Thomas Edison's invention of the light bulb, people slept an average of 10 hours a night; today Americans average 6.9 hours of sleep on weeknights and 7.5 hours per night on weekends."[χ]

A few simple things can help you achieve better sleep and better overall health:

- Avoid caffeine. If you must have your morning coffee, okay, but stay away from caffeine after noontime, as the effects of caffeine can last for up to 12 hours.
- Avoid alcohol too close to bedtime. It may seem to help you get to sleep, but you will often wake up after a few hours, which disrupts the overall sleep pattern you need in order to get the most benefit from sleep.
- Avoid nicotine. It is a stimulant and, by now, you must know how many aspects of your health it's bad for.

[β] "The Benefits of Vitamin C," by Kathleen M. Zelma, *WebMD*, http://www.webmd.com/diet/features/the-benefits-of-vitamin-c.
[χ] "The Sleep Solution Workbook," by G. Frank Lawlis, *Dr. Phil*, http://www.drphil.com/assets/c/c0f3ab7356c5913f1a91dc7c7c347ecc.pdf.

- Avoid eating large meals late at night. Allow enough time to digest your dinner before going to bed.
- Establish good sleep routines. Going to bed at the same time each night can help set your circadian rhythm (your body's internal clock) to help you fall asleep.
- Keep your room cool and dark. Studies suggest that the backlight from devices like laptops, iPads, and televisions can suppress melatonin, which is a natural sleep-inducing hormone.

If you are having trouble, try a natural remedy, like melatonin or chamomile tea, at bedtime. Avoid prescription drugs to help you sleep. They often have adverse effects, such as feeling "hung over" the next morning, and causing a general feeling of fogginess and depression. It is very easy to become dependent on these drugs. If you do, you will be unable to get to sleep without them, and withdrawal from them can be extremely difficult.

THE BENEFITS OF PROPER HYDRATION

Our bodies are made up of mostly water. Muscle tissue is 75% water. Brain tissue is 90% water. Bone tissue is 22% water. Blood is 83% water. Water is vital for every function in the body. Every cell in your body, from head to toe, needs water to:

- Transport nutrients and oxygen into cells
- Moisturize the air in lungs
- Help with metabolism
- Protect our vital organs
- Help our organs to absorb nutrients better
- Regulate body temperature
- Detoxify
- Protect and moisturize our joints

Some of the harmful effects of dehydration I see frequently in patients include tiredness, migraines, constipation, muscle cramps, irregular blood pressure, kidney problems, and dry skin.

In daily life, many people are 1–2% dehydrated. At 5–6% water loss, one may become groggy or sleepy. "With 10% to 15% fluid loss, muscles may become spastic, skin may shrivel and wrinkle, vision may dim, urination will be greatly reduced and may become painful, and delirium may begin. Losses greater than 15% are usually fatal."[7]

The most obvious sign that you are becoming dehydrated is thirst, but it is also one of the later signs. If you are thirsty, you have already gone too long without replenishing your water supply. Earlier signs include dark urine, dry skin, and fatigue.

- Urine: when you are adequately hydrated, your urine should be pale yellow to clear and with only a light odor. If your urine is dark yellow or orange color, or has a strong smell, drink water.
- Skin: your skin is the largest organ you have, and it is your immune system's first line of defense. It requires plenty of water to function properly. If your skin is dry, drink water.
- Fatigue: many people assume fatigue is always a sign that they need sleep or they're hungry, but fatigue is often a sign of dehydration. If you feel tired all the time, drink water.

For many years, it was believed that everyone should drink 8 to 10 glasses of water per day over and above any other liquid. It's not known exactly where this information originated, but it is known now that it was false. While it's certainly a good idea to aim for 8 to 10 eight-ounce glasses or cups of some liquid per day, it's now generally agreed that can include milk, juice, coffee, tea, broth, and even wine and beer. However, it is important to take the impacts of caffeine, sugar, and alcohol on your body, and ensure that water comprises a significant portion of the liquid you drink every day.

---

[7] "Dehydration," Wikipedia, http://en.wikipedia.org/wiki/Dehydration.

CHAPTER **24**:
TAKE CONTROL OF YOUR CHILD'S HEALTH

There's a friend I've referred to a couple of times in this book – the one in the first chapter with the daughter who hated learning about the Industrial Revolution, and again in Chapter 21 where she described her own experiences of food intolerances. The following story is in her words:

I grew up in an interesting family, health-wise. My mother was a registered nurse and believed only in allopathic care, while my father saw a chiropractor long before it was trendy. My mother accepted his use of 'quackery,' as she called it, as long as he didn't expose the children to it.

But in reality, back in the 1960s, they both used many home remedies that would be considered 'alternative' today, like hot lemonade with honey for a cold or vinegar on a canker sore. Although my mother baked a lot, usually with white flour and sugar, she bought few convenience foods, making most things from 'scratch.'

As a result, I grew up with more openness to interesting ideas about health than most children, so, in my twenties, when I had back problems, it wasn't a big leap for me to try a chiropractor. She not only helped with the back issue, but several other issues that had been plaguing me, despite other treatments. And when my second baby had intractable colic every evening at 7 PM, the chiropractor (I'd made an appointment for myself, not my newborn) did an infinitesimally small movement on her tiny body, and the colic never returned.

She was my second child. I'd begun to realize all was not well with my first child's health when he was just six months old and vomiting every time he had a bottle. We soon realized it was a problem with cow's milk. At eight months, he was hospitalized with asthma. By 17 months, he was diagnosed with a whole range of food allergies and he was in hospital almost monthly. Then when my second child was about a year old, her allergy and asthma problems started.

The children's food allergies were tricky because, although they had some allergies in common, they also had many different ones. Trying to make meals we could all eat, and on a tight budget, wasn't easy. The frequent hospitalizations were disruptive, and the asthma drugs made the kids so wired it was like giving them 17 cups of coffee every two hours – their behaviour went wild.

In the meantime, our chiropractor had introduced us to a lot of information about naturopathy and she ultimately 'switched licenses' to practise as an ND. We never abandoned allopathic care; when one of them had an asthma attack, they needed those drugs to breathe, but it became our goal to keep them out of the hospital and off drugs as much as possible with naturopathy.

I did my research and gave my kids various supplements every day. Essential fatty acids cleared up my son's persistent eczema in a few days. Suddenly, I understood why the pediatric dermatologist I'd seen as a child had recommended oatmeal baths for my persistent rash, combined with cortisone cream to control the itching. Back in the 1960s, many allopaths recommended the same combinations of home remedies and prescription drugs that NDs prescribe today.

I also gave my children calcium. Cow's milk made them vomit, one had anaphylaxis to salmon, and the other had anaphylaxis to almonds, so they had no good sources of calcium in their diet. I also gave them vitamin C, to support their immune systems against the asthma attacks.

When they started school, they were the poster children for allergies and asthma. Ironically, though, in spite of their health issues, they always seemed to be the healthiest kids in the school. Their classmates missed a week or two of school a couple of times every year with whatever virus was 'going around.' But once we got past the regular hospital runs in their infancy and learned how to provide integrated care, they rarely got sick.

What my friend describes is a feeling parents often have when their children are so sick they need drugs and hospitals regularly, a feeling of being out of control. Her decision to pursue integrated care allowed her take back that control.

EVALUATE YOUR CHILD'S BODY COMPOSITION

Particularly in an age where children are not learning healthy eating and exercise habits, evaluating body composition is a first step toward understanding any chronic health issues they may be developing. As with adults, many different shapes and sizes fall within the range of normal physical development, but just as you would be concerned if your child showed signs of abnormal mental development, you should be concerned about any tendencies your child shows toward weight issues.

When your child is young, a few extra pounds may seem like no big deal, but if your child has added those pounds as a result of bad health habits, those few pounds can put her at risk for a lifetime of health issues. Allopathic doctors are diagnosing Type II diabetes, intestinal issues, and even high blood pressure in younger and younger children. Childhood obesity is rampant. Ensuring your child is learning good eating and exercise habits is as much an aspect of good parenting as is ensuring they are developing good work habits at school and good social skills with peers.

As your child grows into adolescence, you will notice his food consumption increasing. This is true for both boys and girls, but more so for boys whose muscle mass demands higher caloric input. In fact, many adolescent children can safely eat 3,000 to 4,000 calories a day because their metabolism is very high and they burn those calories off. As they age, however, their metabolism will slow down and their lifestyle will include less daily activity.

If they have developed bad eating habits earlier in life, such as eating large portions, including a lot of junk food in their diets, and spending most of their free time watching television or playing video games, they will likely carry those bad habits into adulthood. They will gain weight and steadily increase their own risk factors for chronic disease. But, if they establish good habits during childhood and adolescence by eating nutritious food, adjusting portion size to their needs for fuel, and incorporating exercise in their daily lives, they will likely reduce their food intake as their energy needs diminish, and remain healthy as they mature into adulthood.

THE BMI FOR CHILDREN AND TEENS

When I evaluate a child's body composition, I begin by calculating body-mass index (BMI) and comparing it to a growth chart for children. As discussed in Chapter 12, BMI often provides unreliable results because it doesn't account for a broad range of body types, but the waist-to-hips (female) and waist-to-chest (male) ratios that I use with adults don't work with children's bodies, because they don't develop in the hips or chest until puberty. For children, the BMI is the best option.

The BMI measures a person's thickness or thinness on a numerical scale. In adults, a BMI of 18.5 to 25 is normal. Anything over 25 is overweight, and anything over 30 is obese, while anything below 18.5 is underweight.* The important thing is to keep weight within a healthy range for age, and BMI charts for children provide a way to measure that.

There are different ways to calculate BMI. It's easy to find BMI calculators online that do the math for you, but it's not difficult to do it yourself. Here's how:

1. Measure your child's height in inches.
2. Calculate the square of your child's height in inches (multiply it by itself). For example, if your child is 4'10" tall, that would be 58 inches. Now multiply 58 X 58 for a result of 3364.
3. Take your child's weight in pounds.
4. Multiply your child's weight by 703. For example, if your child weighs 100 lbs, multiply 100 X 703 for a result of 70,300.
5. Now divide the result of step 4 by the result of step 3. In the example above, you would divide 70,300 by 3364 for a result of 20.89.*

The result of this equation is your child's BMI. You can now compare this to an online chart that shows standard values for

---

* To calculate a BMI using metric measures, you would divide your child's weight in kilograms by the square of the height in centimetres. You would skip step 4, as that is a way of converting imperial to metric. From http://www.wikihow.com/Calculate-BMI-for-Children.

weight and height for children of different ages, and see where your child fits. The Wikipedia page for "Body Mass Index" includes charts for both adults and children, along with the following comments:

> Instead of set thresholds for underweight and overweight, then, the BMI percentile allows comparison with children of the same sex and age. A BMI that is less than the 5th percentile is considered underweight and above the 95th percentile is considered obese for people 20 and under. People under 20 with a BMI between the 85th and 95th percentile are considered to be overweight. Recent studies in Britain have indicated that females between the ages 12 and 16 have a higher BMI than males of the same age by 1.0 kg/m² on average.†

TAKE CONTROL OF YOUR CHILD'S BODY COMPOSITION

If you find your child is becoming heavy, there is no time like the present to take action. By "take action," I don't mean putting your child on a restrictive diet. Children need adequate nutrition as they grow, and forcing any issue around food is likely to backfire and could lead to disordered eating. This is the exact opposite of what children need. Remember that children are like little sponges, soaking up everything they see and hear. You're more likely to be successful with them if you do what you want them to do, than if you tell them to do one thing while you do something different.

Ensure they're eating a healthy breakfast by taking the time to eat with them. Teach them good portioning habits by filling their plates half full with vegetables and dividing the other half between protein and carbohydrates. Buy smaller plates. Put a jug of cold water (not juice) on the table. Encourage kids to chew well and eat slowly. Tell them to wait at least two minutes after their plate is empty before deciding whether they want a second helping.

Think about the kinds of foods you're offering for lunch and dinner. Focus on fresh, unprocessed foods. Take kids along when you go shopping. Let them choose things they like, but steer them toward healthy choices. Involve them in cooking meals. Allow them to share

---

† "Body Mass Index," Wikipedia, http://en.wikipedia.org/wiki/Body_mass_index.

their culinary talents with the family. Make mealtimes occasions to sit down and enjoy each other's company.

What about snack foods? Instead of filling your cupboards with chips, cheesies, and soda pop, make lots of fruit, veggies and dip, crackers and cheese, and yogurt available. If you're all finding it hard to kick the sugar habit, try setting aside one or two days a week when everyone is allowed to have one or two self-indulgent treats. That way, when the kids are asking for junk food, you can remind them (and yourself) to remember what they've asked for when "treat day" comes.

What if I have moments of weakness and find it hard to cut junk foods out of our daily diet?

Remember, you're the one who has to stay strong and provide a good role model. When you feel your resolve weakening, I recommend you review the information in Chapter 4 about the addictive properties of refined sugar, fats, and salt. You wouldn't want your children growing up addicted to drugs, so why would you want them growing up addicted to white sugar and trans-fats?

MAKE EXERCISE FUN

The other important consideration in body composition is exercise. Children don't respond well to the idea of structured workouts, but they love to have fun. If they're having fun, especially with family or friends, they won't notice they're getting exercise. Start by looking over your children's weekly schedules. Are they packed with lessons and team sports? Structured activities are good for children, but it's also good to give them time for unstructured play, especially if it involves going outside and getting fresh air.

When I was growing up in the 1960s, we played outside all the time. Television was new and video games hadn't been imagined yet. We played tag, hide-and-seek, and impromptu games of baseball. We played in the snow and even, if we were dressed for it, in the rain. One of the downsides of filling every minute of your children's time with scheduled activities is that, when nothing is planned, they don't know what to do, so they resort to something electronic.

Several studies have shown that electronics have the same addictive hold over today's children, youth, and young adults as compulsive behaviours like gambling – and internet activity can be just as hard to "kick" as any other addiction. I think about electronics the same way I think about sweets: a bit of self-indulgence is fine, but childhood is the time for your kids to learn healthy habits for maintaining good body composition by having opportunities to use their imaginations in unstructured play with other kids.

It's also important for your children to enjoy healthy, physical activities with you, not by going to aerobics classes or the gym with you (although they may want to do that as they get older), but by walking to and from school with you, going for family bike rides on a sunny weekend, or lacing up the skates for an afternoon of winter fun.

In fact, ensuring that your children are spending plenty of time in a combination of unstructured play with friends, healthy family fun, and an appropriate number of structured activities is one of the best ways you can help them develop good health habits, not only for body composition but for stress management. Remember, the harmful effects of stress come from cortisol building up in your body. When children experience stress and lack opportunities to work it off, cortisol can build up, behavioural issues can arise, and body composition problems can make matters worse.

Even though I've found it impossible to do a formal stress evaluation with children, I can say with certainty that teaching them to get away from the TV and video games and get regular exercise is one of the best ways you can help them develop good habits for body composition and stress management at the same time.

EVALUATE YOUR CHILD'S FOOD INTOLERANCES

If your child's body composition is within the normal range, or if it is outside the normal range but you are taking steps in the right direction, you can move on to testing for food intolerances. I do this very much the same way with children as with adults:

- I perform blood tests to identify possible food intolerances.
- I recommend eliminating all identified foods from the child's diet until symptoms resolve.

- I recommend reintroducing foods one at a time for three days, up to three times a day.
- If symptoms do not return, I recommend trying the next food on the list for three days.
- If a problem occurs, I recommend removing the food from the child's diet, waiting a day or two for the child's system to settle down, and try the next food for three days, up to three times a day.
- Any time problems occur, I remind parents these are their signs to eliminate the most recently added food from their child's diet on an ongoing basis.
- If an intolerance seems confusing (because it shows up some times but not others, for example), I suggest introducing a food twice to rule out false positives.

ADJUST EVALUATION METHODS TO YOUR CHILD'S AGE

If you have an older child or teenager, you may be able to play "food detective" with your child in much the same way you would for yourself. Start by using a food diary to record everything your child eats and asking them to describe any symptoms they experience throughout the day. It can take time for symptoms to show up, so initially you may have to check in with your child 20 or 30 minutes after each meal, then an hour or two later, and again right before the next time they eat.

Keep in mind that all children, even teens, may be reluctant to tell you anything that could mean they'll miss out on something they like, even if it's hurting them; it's up to you to be patient and persistent. With teens in particular, you sometimes have to let them experience discomfort until they're uncomfortable enough to cooperate with you.

The younger the child, the more you will have to adapt your approach to their age and stage of development. For example, if your child is in school but not yet a teenager, he may be old enough to help you verbally with your sleuthing but not to find words to describe the way he feels. You may have to prompt him with questions like, "Does your tummy hurt? Can you show me where? Is it a sharp pain, like a knife? Or is it more like cramps, like before you go to the bathroom? Do you feel like you need to burp a lot, or like you might throw up?"

With infants, toddlers, and even preschoolers, you may have to rely on observation. Does your child throw up in relation to any food? Does any food seem related to bouts with diarrhea or constipation? Do your child's feces change colour (usually a greenish colour indicates some sort of digestive upset)? Is your child colicky, or burping more than usual? Has a skin rash come up? If so, where is it, and what does it look like? Does your child ever have mood swings, or temper tantrums? All young children can have mercurial temperaments, but parents are usually the most likely to know when their mood changes are out of the ordinary.

Write it all down in the food diary – all the foods, all the symptoms, and any behaviour that seems out of the ordinary. They may not all mean something, but you won't find the ones that are meaningful unless you write everything down and review it for patterns and relationships.

TAKE CONTROL OF YOUR CHILD'S FOOD INTOLERANCES

Once you've identified a list of possible offending foods, you'll need to proceed in much the same way as I described for adults. First, withdraw the foods you've identified for about three weeks to ensure your child's body is clear of symptoms. Then begin re-introducing foods one at a time, up to three times a day, for three days.

If the child is clear of symptoms after three days, introduce the next food. If your child has immediate and severe symptoms, like vomiting within minutes of eating the food, you may want to withdraw it without trying it again. If the symptoms are milder or take longer to surface, such as a skin rash, you may wish to persist for up to three days to confirm the relationship. If you have concerns about false positives, you may wish to withdraw the food and try again another time.

Before you try again, you may want to teach yourself the fine art of label reading. If your child is reacting to a single food, like eggs or strawberries, the results of your testing are probably reliable, but if the food causing the reaction contains several ingredients, you may have to experiment to determine which one is causing the problem – or if it's more than one.

For example, if your child throws up after eating waffles, is he reacting to the flour, eggs, milk, or one of the toppings? The food diary will probably give you a good idea of where to start. So rather than subjecting her to an unpleasant test with a food you think is problematic, try testing the foods you think are less likely to be causing the reaction. The allergy may be simpler to manage than you feared; you may find one or more of the other foods also cause reactions; or you may find several foods are causing similar reactions and your child needs to avoid them all.

Even if the intolerance seems simple, it may not be. If your child reacts to cow's milk, for example, it could be a response to the protein, the fat, or the sugar. If she/he reacts to the sugar (lactose), the solution may be as simple as buying milk with the enzyme lactase added.

Don't be too quick to jump to conclusions. If your child seems to be reacting to blueberries, she might actually be reacting to sulphites sprayed on the berries to prevent mould. Try washing your fruit with a gentle produce wash, or buying organically grown berries from a source you trust.

Diagnosing your child's food intolerances can be a long and tedious process. It is quicker and easier to start with blood testing, but if you are unable to see a naturopath, an elimination diet followed by a series of food challenges (which is what I've been describing) is the best way to do it on your own. And again, although I don't assess children directly for stress, I can say with certainty that eating foods that make them feel bad causes their bodies to feel stress. Even though it may be difficult to coax them through diagnosis of food intolerances and to get them used to the idea of eating alternatives, in the long run, it will also reduce their stress levels.

TOXIC LOAD: A SPECIAL CONCERN FOR CHILDREN

In Chapters 7, 14, and 23, I provided information about organic and inorganic toxins, how they get into our food, air, and water, how they accumulate in our bodies, and what detoxification processes I use to help patients reduce their toxic load.

Toxic load is of particular concern to children because they are significantly more susceptible to toxic exposure than adults. This is partly because their bodies are smaller and their threshold for a toxic response is much lower; but more importantly, it's because children's bodies are still developing and toxic build-up can interfere with their development.

This is of particular concern to brain development. A 2014 study published in the medical journal *The Lancet Neurology* listed 11 organic and inorganic toxins of serious concern to children's brain development. The 11 toxins include many I've mentioned in earlier chapters, and several more. Most industrial nations have already banned these chemicals, but they are still in use in some poorer nations.

The list includes several toxins listed in Chapters 7 and 23: lead, mercury, polychlorinated biphenyls (PCBs), brominated flame retardants (PBDEs), bisphenol-A (BPA), and phthalates. For more information on the impacts of these toxins, please review earlier information. In addition, the authors of *The Lancet Neurology* article have identified another six of growing concern:

- Arsenic: studies have linked arsenic in drinking water with reduced *cognitive* (thinking) function in school-age kids.
- Toluene: being exposed to this solvent during pregnancy can cause brain development problems and attention deficit in the child.
- Manganese: though this mineral is important in trace amounts, studies have linked high levels in drinking water with lower scores in math, poor intellectual function, and ADHD.
- Fluoride: high levels of fluoride (the same stuff your dentist puts on your child's teeth) has been linked with lower IQs in children.
- Chlorpyrifos and DDT (pesticides): these have been linked with structural abnormalities in the brain. Though banned in many countries, they are still used in some parts of the developing world.

- Tetrachloroethylene (AKAperchlorethylene): hyperactivity, aggressive behavior, and psychiatric issues are some of the problems connected with this chemical. Women who work as nurses, chemists, cleaners, hairdressers, and beauticians are often exposed.

At levels of exposure so low they would have no effect on adults, all of these toxins can lead to permanent brain damage in children, causing them to suffer "reduced attention span, delayed development, and poor school performance."[‡] Yet avoiding these chemicals can be difficult because they are present in almost everything we touch. Plastic food containers, children's furniture and toys, outdoor furniture, vinyl window blinds, non-stick cookware, children's clothing, carpets and furniture, deodorant, hand lotions, and cosmetics, paints, cleaning solutions, and foods that have absorbed pesticides – it's hard to think of anything in the world around us that isn't laced with toxins.

WHAT CAN YOU DO ABOUT YOUR CHILD'S TOXIC LOAD?

Various websites, such as the Environmental Working Group's Dirty Dozen Endocrine Disruptors and Dr. Joseph Mercola's website, offer ideas on how to help your family avoid toxic build-up, but if it's already occurred, what do you do? I recommend the same thing for children as for adults: if you have done as much as you can to work through the algorithm on your own but your child is still having symptoms, find a naturopathic doctor to evaluate for toxic load and recommend a detoxification protocol.

I test for toxic load in children in much the same way as in adults, and use similar treatment protocols. As I've said, in my clinic, I test only for inorganic toxins, like lead and mercury, but you can check with your local or national naturopathic association for a naturopathic doctor near you who is familiar with organic toxins. Please see Chapter 23 for information on how to find a naturopathic doctor and assess his or her credentials. Remember, you are looking

---

[‡] "11 Toxic Chemical Affecting Brain Development in Children," by Alice G. Walton, Forbes, Feb 15, 2014, http://www.forbes.com/sites/alicegwalton/2014/02/15/11-toxic-chemicals-afffecting-brain-development-in-children/.

for a professional who uses the designation ND or NMD. If you find someone who simply calls himself a "naturopath," stay away.

SLEEP AND YOUR CHILD

Like adults, children and youth need sleep and water for wellness. But where the average adult needs seven to eight hours sleep per night, children and youth need much more. In the first year of life, infants need up to 16 hours of sleep per day. From one to three years, the requirement drops to 12–14 hours, and then to 10–12 hours from three to six years of age. It continues dropping as children get older, with 7- to 12-year-olds needing about 10–11 hours, and 12- to 18-year-olds needing 9–10 hours.

Teenagers are legendary for their ability to sleep late, and to be difficult to rouse. During adolescence, youth have much longer cycles of deep-wave sleep. It's what their growing bodies and brains need for good health, development, and performance. According to the Sleep Foundation:

> The consequences of sleep deprivation during the teenage years are particularly serious. Teens spend a great portion of each day in school; however, they are unable to maximize the learning opportunities afforded by the education system, since sleep deprivation impairs their ability to be alert, pay attention, solve problems, cope with stress and retain information. Young people who do not get enough sleep night after night carry a significant risk for drowsy driving; emotional and behavioural problems such as irritability, depression, poor impulse control and violence; health complaints; tobacco and alcohol use; impaired cognitive function and decision-making; and lower overall performance in everything from academics to athletics.[δ]

Sleep is not a luxury for children and youth. Particularly in the upper grades of high school and early post-secondary education, youth need their sleep to avoid accidental injury and make the most

---

[δ] "Backgrounder: Later School Start Times," National Sleep Foundation, http://sleepfoundation.org/sleep-news/backgrounder-later-school-start-times.

of whatever training they're undertaking in preparation for adult life. Sleeping away the whole day and throwing their bodies off a sensible sleep-wake cycle is not a good idea. However, for the most part, parents should cut teenagers some slack around sleeping. Soon enough, they'll be adults with children of their own and they'll learn what sleep deprivation is really all about!

WATER AND YOUR CHILD

Similarly, I can't stress enough that children are more susceptible than adults to dehydration, for several reasons. Proportionally, children have more body surface area than adults, so they heat up more quickly; because their movements are less efficient, they generate more heat during similar activities. Also, children's sweating mechanisms are not as mature as adults', so they do not cool off as efficiently; and children who are overweight tend to heat up more quickly, and are at even greater risk of dehydration than their peers.

The fact is that children need to learn to drink lots of water. Studies show children often drink less plain water than they really should. It's not that they don't get thirsty but that they don't find water appealing when they're being offered so many sweet options, like fruit juice and carbonated beverages. But too much sugar exacerbates dehydration and packs on calories. Diluting fruit juice can make drinking a little more fun for kids. You might try having a jug of cold water on the table to sip with meals while reserving diluted fruit juice for snack times.

Once again, although I don't assess stress directly in children, ensuring they are getting adequate sleep and drinking enough plain water is bound to reduce their stress levels. More importantly, it helps them learn good health habits from the time they're young. As they mature, those good habits will become second nature. And remember, good habits are just as hard to break as bad ones. When you take control of your child's body composition, food intolerances, and toxic load, you will teach them, by example, how to take responsibility for their health by taking every possible step to prevent illness. You will be practising Generational Health First. I'll talk more about that in the final chapter.

CHAPTER 25:
TAKE CONTROL OF HEALTH CARE

Many years ago a middle-aged woman came to see me. She had a late-life child, a daughter of about three years, so she had been looking forward to a long and healthy future, and she had every reason to expect it. She had no previous personal or family history of serious illness and she had no history of taking drugs, whether prescription or recreational.

The only issue she'd ever had was with heavy menses that lasted about a week. That, in itself, was not unusual, and if she had come to see me before seeing an allopathic physician, I would have had no reason to recommend preventive measures against anything.

Yet she had recently been diagnosed with uterine cancer. She'd had a hysterectomy, the cancer appeared to have been fully removed, and there seemed to be no metastasis (spreading to other tissues). She'd been dismissed with no recommendations other than regular follow-ups. She had come to me for support in recovering from a surgery that threw her hormones out of balance and plunged her into menopause. I treated her for a while, and then didn't see her for several years.

Seven years after she'd been declared cancer-free, a routine follow-up with her oncologist revealed a malignant neoplasm (abnormal growth) in the bone tissue in her lower back. She now faced a battle with chemotherapy and radiation. Her prognosis was not good. There was not much I could do for her. I wondered, what was the purpose of those routine follow-ups if not to provide her with some advice that might have been truly preventive in nature? Was their only purpose early diagnosis of another lesion? In this case, by the time diagnosis happened, it was too late.

Having been given a clean bill of health by her allopathic doctors, and having used my advice to manage the dramatic effects of surgical menopause, she'd left my care confident that the cancer was gone and the follow-up checks would suffice to ensure her continued good health.

There is, of course, no way of knowing whether I could have helped her prevent her second, fatal bout with cancer, but I do know that if she'd continued in my care, integrating the expertise of allopathic and naturopathic approaches, my strategy would have been very different than it was. If I'd had the chance after her surgery succeeded to do more than manage her surgical menopause, I would have reviewed her personal and family history more deeply. The fact that she seemed healthy to begin with yet developed cancer anyway would have been reason enough for me to dig deeper.

I would have asked if there were any racial or ethnic predispositions in her background. I would have asked about her living conditions as a child, whether she'd grown up poor and perhaps suffered dietary deficiencies. I would have reviewed her exercise routines, checked for undiagnosed food intolerances, analysed her stress management habits. I would have wanted to know about her occupational and geographic history so I could assess exposure to organic or inorganic toxins. I would have checked typical parameters of wellness to see if her body was, in fact, aging more quickly than it appeared to be. There was actually a great deal more I could have done that might have been better than taking a wait-and-see approach.

There is no way to know whether anyone might have done anything to help this patient remain cancer free. However, I do know that I have patients for whom I have done in-depth cancer follow-ups, patients who have followed my guidelines, and who remain cancer free. Was it my recommendations that helped? I'll never know, but I don't think my patients care. The only thing that matters to them is that they're alive, they're healthy, and they have more time to share the gift of health with everyone they love.

TRUE PREVENTION VS EARLY DETECTION

In my experience, many people confuse prevention with early detection. What allopathic doctors offered to the woman in the preceding story was early detection, which unfortunately was not early enough. What naturopathic doctors strive to provide is prevention, which involves reading the signs of risk and taking steps to prevent it from progressing into disease.

Prevention seems like such a common sense idea, but within the boundaries of allopathic medicine, it's difficult to put into practice. Allopathic medicine is based on science. Science is about proving things in a way we can see. If a person gets sick, and they take a drug and they get well, we can see that. We can prove the drug worked.

It's more difficult to prove naturopathic methods work. We detect biomarkers that allopathic medicine doesn't typically measure, or at least not for the same purposes. We provide treatments that allopathic medicine doesn't accept, because it's hard to test them using allopathic research methods. We try to prevent disease from developing, but how do we prove prevention? Proving naturopathic medicine works isn't easy, at least not using allopathic methods, and allopathic methods are considered the gold standard, the bar that all other health care disciplines have to reach for.

That's slowly changing. People are becoming increasingly aware that statements made by allopathic doctors 30 years ago were not quite as well proved as we once thought. Consider the arguments my classmates and I had about antibiotics with allopathic medical students back in the 1980s. We had it right; they had it wrong. Consider the massive public health campaign against fats, based on allopathic research that fats were the root of heart disease. Again, we had it right; they had it wrong.

I could offer many other examples, but my point is not to suggest that naturopathic medicine is all good and allopathic medicine is all bad. As I described in the Introduction to the book, much of the animosity between our two disciplines in the early years of naturopathy was our own fault. As I also described, we made some grave mistakes and saw a few patients suffer tragic losses. Allopathic medicine has had its share of mistakes, too. As I've said throughout the book, it's not an us-and-them situation, or at least it shouldn't be, because both disciplines work better when they work together.

SAVING LIVES AND SAVING DOLLARS

Throughout this book, I've been describing where naturopathic medicine fits in individual health care. But it's just as important to take a broad overview and see where naturopathic medicine fits into our culture. Preventive medicine fits into a full spectrum of health care not only because it saves costs in human suffering, but because it saves costs in dollars and cents.

Just as Dr. Jheeta's Algorithm can help patients take control of their health, naturopathic medicine can help all of us take control of our health care system. A recent fact sheet published by the American Association of Naturopathic Physicians supports this. I quote it in its entirety:

> Numerous studies have demonstrated that using non-invasive, non-toxic approaches lowers health care costs. Patients with the greatest disease burden show the most significant reduction in total medical expenditures when utilizing integrative medicine. Fifty-five percent of patients reported a slight to substantial reduction of their use of conventional medical care once they begin visiting an integrative medicine provider. A systematic review of randomized clinical trials found that use of natural health products has the potential to reduce costs of conventional treatment by up to 73%.
>
> Naturopathic approaches to reducing cardiovascular disease risk factors, such as hypertension and high cholesterol, and symptoms of menopause save money. Many studies have also documented cost savings resulting from use of naturopathic physicians to reduce pain, especially back pain...
>
> Many studies have found that naturopathic care results in substantially lower prescription drug costs than conventional care. Naturopathic physicians typically prescribe botanical or nutritional supplements to effectively care for medical problems rather than expensive prescription drugs. Patients who received intensive lifestyle modification and naturopathic therapy in just one year for type II diabetes improved all health scores (lipid levels, body

fat percentage, etc.) and decreased medication requirements compared to those on standard therapy. Integrative medicine users in two studies reported significantly lower prescription drug use of 48% and 61%, respectively...

By addressing the causes of disease, naturopathic physicians reduce the need for repeated, expensive and often ineffective symptomatic treatment. A study published in JAMA found that patients of integrative medicine providers were significantly more likely to have obtained common preventive services, including pap smears, cholesterol testing, influenza immunizations, and breast exams...

A recent study found that patients receiving one year of care under the supervision of a naturopathic doctor experienced a 3.1% reduction in 10-year CVD event risk compared to patients receiving conventional care. They were also 16.9% less likely to have developed metabolic syndrome. This resulted in significant savings to society of $1,138 per patient and to employers of $1,167...

Studies of insurance costs provide strong evidence that including naturopathic physicians saves money. One study of special note demonstrates that the majority of patient visits to naturopathic physicians are in lieu of – not in addition to – conventional medical care. Studies have found the per visit expenditures to integrative medicine providers cost only 52% as much for conventional outpatient care and that annual expenditures for insured integrative medicine users in Washington State were $356 less than for non-integrative medicine users. An internal Blue Shield Study in King County, WA estimated that a naturopathic centered managed care program could cut the costs of chronic and stress related illnesses by up to 40% and lower costs of specialist utilization by up to 30%.[*]

[*] "Naturopathic Medicine Lowers Health Care Costs," Including Naturopathic Physicians in Medicare, American Association of Naturopathic Physicians, http://aanp.membershipsoftware.org/files/About_Naturopathic_Medicine/fact%20sheet%20-%20cost-effectiveness.pdf.
See also "Naturopathic Approaches to High-Cost Diseases," Including Naturopathic Physicians in Medicare, American Association of Naturopathic Physicians,

THE DOCTOR OF THE FUTURE

For the most part, when I speak of making generational health our first priority, I'm speaking to patients, because I believe individual responsibility is where all positive change begins. But, I'm also speaking to my fellow physicians, both naturopathic and allopathic. Medicine can be a very rewarding calling. In this book, I've shared many stories of experiences that have given me a deep sense of fulfillment in knowing I chose the right profession.

But as I look back over 30 years, I also recall the experiences that taught me harder lessons. The young Latina woman who refused to seek allopathic care for her cancer, and the middle-aged woman who, perhaps, I should have pushed a little harder to take a more proactive, preventive approach. I can't help but think that a better-integrated system of health care – a system in which allopathic and naturopathic physicians work together to complement each other's strengths instead of debating each other's weaknesses – might have saved them both.

I'll never know, but I know how hard it is to lose a patient. All doctors know. I believe one of the things the doctor of the future will do is integrate the naturopathic and allopathic sides of health care better so as to reduce the number of patients we have to let go of, to reduce the number of times we have to think "If only I could have done this ..." or "If only my patient had done that ..."

We will never prevent every death, we will never prevent every illness, or every accident, and we will always need allopathic medicine, but we need naturopathic medicine, too. The chronic illnesses that comprise such a large portion of our health expenditures today do not need to happen as often as they do, much less as often as they are projected to do in the coming years. Look back at the World Health Organization's numbers provided in the Introduction to the book. They are as frightening because of what they mean for the cost of health care in dollars as for what they mean for the cost in human suffering. But they don't have to be.

---

http://aanp.membershipsoftware.org/files/About_Naturopathic_Medicine/fact%20sheet%20-%20naturopathic%20modalities.pdf.

If naturopathic doctors and allopathic doctors worked together to provide a broader spectrum of care than either can alone, I believe we could reduce human suffering, reduce the financial costs of health care, and take back control of health and our health care system. I believe the doctor of the future will do this: she will integrate allopathic and naturopathic skills so seamlessly that neither she nor her patients will know where one ends and the other begins, and that is as it should be. Just as there should be no false division between mind and body, there should be no false division between doctors who practice proactive skills and those who practice reactive skills. Both are needed to build a health care discipline that covers the full spectrum of care.

RESPONDING TO CRISIS WITH PREVENTION

I feel such a strong sense of urgency about getting my message out, and sharing my vision. Our health care system is in crisis. Costs are spiralling out of control. I fear for the number of patients who may be left behind because we have not moved quickly enough in the direction of integrating our practices and envisioning together the kind of care the doctor of the future will provide: care that focuses first on prevention, with the skills for reaction when it's appropriate; care that sees an emergency and leaps into action; care that focuses on making generational health our first priority as much as it should be our patients' first priority.

I know I sound like an idealist, but I hope I sound like a realist, too. My sense of urgency comes partly from knowing there is a long road ahead, and the sooner we take the first step, the sooner we will arrive at our destination. It could be an arduous journey. There will be many disagreements along the way, but I believe it's a worthwhile road to travel. Because at the end of the road I call Generational Health First, there is a wonderful gift, a gift we can all share, a gift we can give ourselves, our children, and each other. It's the gift of health. There is no better gift we can give or receive, and there is no better time to set out on the journey towards that gift than right now.

CONCLUSION

Some years ago, a man of 47 years came into the clinic. He was overweight, had low energy but high blood pressure, and he felt anxious, restless, and depressed much of the time. He wasn't sleeping well and said he couldn't taste or smell his food properly. He had a family medical history that included many instances of heart disease, cancer, and arthritis, but when I asked whether he was using this awareness to decrease his risk of developing those diseases, his answer suggested resignation.

"I was taught to believe these things are in God's hands," he said.

"So what's changed that's brought you here now?" I asked.

"Well," he said, "I've watched so many people I loved wait to find out what God had in store for them. And then once they had a heart attack or found a lump, they took it on faith that it was part of God's plan for them. I've watched people I loved slowly deteriorate and die."

"But lately," he continued, "I've started wondering: Is it really God's will for us to get ill and die in such a heartbreaking way? Or does God want us to find ways to stay alive, and healthy?"

"I'm not qualified to answer those questions," I said. "But I am qualified to help you figure out if there are ways to assess your risk factors and reduce your risk of developing one of those serious illnesses that seem to run in your family."

He agreed, and on a hunch I decided that, rather than following the algorithm as usual, I would take a more functional approach with this patient – I would test for how healthy he was instead of how sick he was. I wanted to know how well his body was dealing with stress, processing food, and managing toxic load.

223

I started by testing his urine for cortisol,* his blood for fasting insulin, and his urine for toxic load. His cortisol levels were high regardless of the time of day, his insulin was correspondingly high, and blood tests revealed considerable build-up of lead, mercury, and beryllium. The next time I saw him, I shared these test results and asked more about his stress levels.

"I have a very demanding job," he said. "I have frequent deadlines. It's a constant source of stress. And I was raised to meet expectations."

"I agree that's important," I said. "But I imagine your family has expectations of you, too. And I wonder how well you're going to meet their expectations if you get sick, or you die."

"I don't understand," he said.

"These results tell me that stress is a significant factor in many of your symptoms. Your high cortisol could be causing your feelings of anxiety and difficulty sleeping. It could also be a factor in your weight," I said. "I believe you have an opportunity to act on this now, before any of the diseases that have plagued so many of your loved ones catch up with you."

I prescribed some botanical supplements to help bring his cortisol down, and suggested some lifestyle changes to improve his body composition. I also started him on chelation therapy for the heavy metal build-up, explaining that although the body can eliminate these metals, his family history suggested his body would excrete them much more slowly than most people, and that could be causing some of his symptoms, too.

He began exercising, starting small and building over time. He picked up a hobby to get his mind off stressful issues, and lower his anxiety. He even started taking yoga classes.

"How are you feeling?" I asked on a subsequent visit.

"Good," he said. "I'm sleeping better. I have more energy. Even my food smells and tastes better, so I'm enjoying it more. Yet, as you can see, he said (patting his mid-section), I'm losing weight."

This didn't surprise me. The most recent tests showed his cortisol stabilizing, which was why he was sleeping better and had

---

* I've since changed to blood tests in addition to urinary tests for cortisol, and blood tests to assess toxic load.

more energy. His insulin level and appetite had also stabilized, so he no longer craved sugars and carbohydrates. As the pounds came off, his blood pressure came down.

He continued chelation therapy until the toxins in his blood had returned to acceptable levels. I then wanted to test for his body's ability to neutralize toxins, so I recommended indirect detoxification protocols. During phase 1, his body was able to neutralize toxins to some extent, but during phase 2 it was not able to convert them into water-soluble products to be eliminated in his urine. This was the culprit causing toxic build-up in his body. I prescribed botanical supplements to remedy this.

When I first saw this patient, I think any doctor, allopathic or naturopathic, would have read his family history, seen the biomarkers of disease, and predicted what I predicted – that he was well on his way to obesity, diabetes, hypertension, heart attack, perhaps arthritis, possibly cancer, probably death earlier than necessary.

By the last time I saw this patient, his risk of developing any of these chronic degenerative diseases had been diminished and his overall sense of well-being had improved. He had put his health in the hands of naturopathic medicine, which strives to put it back in the patient's hands. We had worked together proactively to prevent disease instead of waiting until disease could be diagnosed and then acting reactively, with drugs to manage the disease. We had practised prevention instead of palliation.

There is no way of knowing what the final outcome for this patient will be. But beyond his reduced risk of disease and his own overall feeling of wellness, he is now sharing his enthusiasm for naturopathic medicine with those around him. Since I last saw him, he has referred numerous patients to our clinic, or to naturopathic medicine in general. He's actively working to spread awareness that predisposition to disease does not mean it can't be prevented, and that living a healthy lifestyle can transform anyone's life. He is one of the best examples I can remember in all my years of practice of the way people can begin to make Generational Health First a priority, and because of what he learned in the process he has now taken back control of his own health.

MAKE GENERATIONAL HEALTH FIRST YOUR PRIORITY

When I speak of making generational health your first priority, this man is one of many patients I think of. He came from a family that had passed generational ill-health from grandparents to parents to children. When he decided to take control of his health, he changed that and began passing generational good health along to his family, as well as to friends and colleagues.

If you don't take anything else from this book, I hope you will take this one core message. When we take control of our health and make decisions that help us minimize the risk of developing devastating, life-changing diseases, we are not only giving ourselves an immeasurable gift. We are giving our loved ones the greatest gift we can give them. We are giving them more time to spend with us when we are in good health. We are giving them an example of how to bring better health into their own lives. We are showing them a way to pass the gift of good health along to their own children.

This is the meaning of putting Generational Health First.

It is my purpose in this book to share my belief widely that there's nothing more important we can do in life than put Generational Health First. This concept allows us to work hard to support our loved ones, to play and enjoy their company, to stay alive and experience good health together with them for as long as possible. To me, this is an idea whose time has come, an idea to be passed on to our children, and our grandchildren, and our great-grandchildren until it has become a fully accepted fact of life.

Over 30 years ago, I decided to become a naturopathic doctor and, in the decades since then, I've shaped my philosophy of health into my life's mission. That mission is to introduce the idea of generational health first in such a compelling way that people today will see it and think, "Of course! That makes so much sense!" My goal is for so many people to adopt the philosophy of Generational Health First that it will become second nature. My vision is that, a few generations from now, it will be so natural for people to put generational health first that no one will even use the words anymore.

My dream is that one day, one of our great-great-great grandchildren will find a copy of this book in an attic, and they'll take it to their parents and ask, "What does it mean to make generational health your first priority?" Their parents will tell them the meaning of that old-time saying, and the children will say, "Well, that's just normal. Why would it need a special name? Why would anyone think anything else?"

Indeed, why would anyone think anything else?

A FINAL WORD

Naturopathic medicine is still a young discipline, but I believe it has a great deal to offer each of us as individuals, and all of us as communities. I won't dwell on financial issues facing the healthcare system in this book, but I do want to mention here, that I believe the integration of naturopathic medicine into the national healthcare system has the potential not only to reduce human suffering, but to reduce the financial cost of that suffering.

Many people who read this book who are presumed to be reasonably healthy will have immediate benefits and results from using my algorithm. But others who are not in good physical conditions for various reasons must realize that the longer the body has been ignored the longer it may take to return to 100% health. So with that in mind, the speed at which you absorb this knowledge and implement the necessary changes will be a direct factor on how quickly results are achieved.

We can see now that Naturopathic medicine is not the perfect creature I thought it was when I began my education in 1983. It's much more than that. It's a discipline that encompasses many so-called alternative approaches to health care, and one that can fit hand in glove with allopathic medicine to provide a truly full spectrum of health care to patients. I believe the potential for the two disciplines to work together are virtually limitless. Since there are numerous doctors such as myself who have taken this integrative approach, you now know that there are other solutions to your health issues, and the Doctor of the future is here to help.

SOURCES

CHAPTER 1

The information on changes in family farming is from "Canada's Farm Population: Agriculture-Population Linkage Data for the 2006 Census" on *Statistics Canada* at http://www.statcan.gc.ca/ca-ra2006/agpop/article-eng.htm; "Family Farm" on *Wikipedia* at http://en.wikipedia.org/wiki/Family_farm; "Nutritional Differences in Organic versus Conventional Foods: And the Winner Is..." on *Scientific American* at http://blogs.scientificamerican.com/guest-blog/2011/08/11/nutritional-differences-in-organic-vs-conventional-foods-and-the-winner-is/; "Organic Food No More Nutritious Than Conventionally Grown Food" on *Harvard Health Publications* at http://www.health.harvard.edu/blog/organic-food-no-more-nutritious-than-conventionally-grown-food-201209055264; "Nutrition and Healthy Eating" on *Mayo Clinic* at http://www.mayoclinic.com/health/organic-food/NU00255/NSECTIONGROUP=2; and "Is Local More Nutritious? It Depends," on *Harvard Education* at http://chge.med.harvard.edu/sites/default/files/resources/local_nutrition.pdf.

CHAPTER 2

The information on the history of canning came from "Canning" on *Wikipedia* at http://en.wikipedia.org/wiki/Canning.
The information about fast food came from "Fast Food" on *Wikipedia* at http://en.wikipedia.org/wiki/Fast_food; *Fast Food Nation* by Eric Schlosser (Penguin, 2002) at http://jhampton.pbworks.com/w/file/fetch/51769044/Fast%20Food%20Nation.pdf; "Still a Fast-Food Nation: Eric Schlosser Reflects on 10 Years Later" on *The Daily Beast* at http://www.thedailybeast.com/articles/2012/03/12/still-a-fast-food-nation-eric-schlosser-reflects-on-10-years-later.html; "55 Juicy Facts About... Fast Food" on *Random Facts* at http://facts.randomhistory.com/2009/06/27_fast-food.html; and "McDonald's the Holy Grail for Potato Farmers" on *NBC News* at

http://www.nbcnews.com/id/32983108/ns/business-us_business/t/mcdonalds-holy-grail-potato-farmers/.
The information on non-communicable diseases is from *World Health Organization* at
http://www.who.int/mediacentre/factsheets/fs310/en/index1.html and http://apps.who.int/gho/data/node.main.686?lang=en.

CHAPTER 3

The information about the history of the pharmaceutical industry came from "Pfizer's History" on *Pfizer* at
http://www.pfizer.ca/en/about_pfizer/corporate_background/pfizer_history; "Syrette" on *Wikipedia* at
http://en.wikipedia.org/wiki/Syrette; and "History" on *Bristol Myers Squibb* at
http://www.bms.com/ourcompany/Pages/history.aspx.
The information on statin drugs came from "Statin Adverse Effects" on *University of California San Diego* at
https://www.statineffects.com/info/adverse_effects.htm; and "It's Time to Question the New Guidelines on Cholesterol Drugs" by André Picard in *The Globe and Mail*, November 24, 2013 at
http://www.theglobeandmail.com/life/health-and-fitness/health/its-time-to-question-the-new-guidelines-on-cholesterol-drugs/article15566990/.
The information on the University of British Columbia study came from "Doctors Not Informed of Harmful Effects of Medicines during Sales Visits," *UBC Public Affairs*, April 10, 2013 at
http://www.publicaffairs.ubc.ca/2013/04/10/doctors-not-informed-of-harmful-effects-of-medicines-during-sales-visits/.

CHAPTER 4

The information on sugar is from "Sugar Can Be Addictive, Princeton Scientist Says," by Kitta MacPherson, December 10, 2008 on *News at Princeton* at
http://www.princeton.edu/main/news/archive/S22/88/56G31/index.xml?section=topstories; and Dr. Sanjay Gupta, "Sugar," a segment on *60 Minutes*, aired on CNN April 1, 2012 and posted October 29,

2012 as "Sugar Exposé, 60 Minutes, Dr. Sanjay Gupta" on *YouTube* at https://www.youtube.com/watch?v=HezSlrJ1k7w.
The information on fats came from "Sugar and Fat Bingeing Have Notable Differences in Addictive-like Behavior," by Nicole M. Avena, Pedro Rada, and Bartley G. Hoebel in *Journal of Nutrition,* Mar 2009, volume 139, issue 3, pages 623–628, on *PubMed* at http://www.ncbi.nlm.nih.gov/pmc/articles/PMC2714381/; "Not All Trans Fats Are Equally Risky," by Stephanie Watson, *WebMD Health News,* March 7, 2008 at http://www.webmd.com/cholesterol-management/news/20080307/not-all-trans-fats-are-equally-risky; "Trans-fat Diet Induces Abdominal Obesity and Changes in Insulin Sensitivity in Monkeys," by K. Kavanagh, KL Jones, J Sawyer, K Kelley, JJ Carr, JD Wagner, LL Rudel, *Obesity,* July 2007, volume 15, issue 7, pages 1675–84, on *PubMed* at http://www.ncbi.nlm.nih.gov/pubmed/17636085; "Cholesterol Abnormalities & Diabetes," on *American Heart Association* at https://www.heart.org/HEARTORG/Conditions/Diabetes/WhyDiabetesMatters/Cholesterol-Abnormalities-Diabetes_UCM_313868_Article.jsp; "Why Are Trans-Fats Bad for Men's and Women's Fertility?" on *Fertility Health* at http://www.fertility-health.com/why-are-trans-fats-bad.html; "Tip of the Week: Non-Alcoholic Fatty Liver Disease, and How to Cure It," by Steven E. Greer, MD, January 23, 2013 on *Current Medicine* at http://www.currentmedicine.tv/2013/01/23/tip-of-the-week-non-alcoholic-fatty-liver-disease-and-how-to-cure-it/; "Link between Fast Food and Depression Confirmed," March 30, 2012 on *Science Daily* at http://www.sciencedaily.com/releases/2012/03/120330081352.htm; "Saturated Fat Not Bad for You," March 10, 2014 on *Toronto Sun* at http://www.torontosun.com/2014/03/10/saturated-fat-not-bad-for-you; and "Observations: Saturated Fat is not the Major Issue," on *British Medical Journal*, Oct 22, 2013 at http://www.bmj.com/press-releases/2013/10/22/observations-saturated-fat-not-major-issue.
The information on salt came from "Salt and Sodium," *The Nutrition Source*, Harvard School of Public Health at http://www.hsph.harvard.edu/nutritionsource/salt-and-sodium/; "Go Easy on the Salt," by Mara Betsch on *Health* at http://www.health.com/health/gallery/0,,20365078,00.html; "Why

Is There So Much Salt in Processed Foods?" by Brian Palmer, May 15, 2103 on *Slate.com* at http://www.slate.com/articles/health_and_science/explainer/2013/05/salt_dietary_guidelines_why_do_food_manufacturers_use_so_much_salt.html; and "Are You Salt Deficient?" by Dr. David Brownstein, *Caduseus*, issue 79, pages 16–19, at http://www.anh-europe.org/files/David_Brownstein_article_Caduceus_issue_79_Are_you_salt_deficient.pdf.

The information on exercise is from "Physical Exercise," on Wikipedia at http://en.wikipedia.org/wiki/Physical_exercise; and "When Did We Start Getting Fat?" by Roger Highfield on *The Telegraph,* June 6, 2007 at http://www.telegraph.co.uk/science/science-news/3296662/When-DID-we-start-getting-fat.html.

CHAPTER 5

Information on an allopathic view of food allergies and intolerances is from "Disease Summaries: Food Allergy," on *World Allergy Association,* May 2004 at http://www.worldallergy.org/professional/allergic_diseases_center/foodallergy/.

Information on a naturopathic view of food intolerances is from "Food Allergies: 5 Myths Debunked," by Katrina Woznicki on *WebMD* at http://www.webmd.com/allergies/features/food-allergy-myths; and "Food Intolerance" on *Wikipedia* at http://en.wikipedia.org/wiki/Food_intolerance.

Information on refined sugar impacts is from "Junk Food Starts Allergies: Western High-Fat Diets are Blamed for Surge in Illnesses," by David Derbyshire, *Daily Mail,* August 3, 2010 at http://www.dailymail.co.uk/health/article-1299805/Junk-food-starts-allergies-Western-high-fat-diets-blamed-surge-illnesses.html#ixzz33APHVJP9; and "Study: Severe Food Allergies More Common Among Children," by Jason Kane on *The Rundown on PBS Newshour,* June 20, 2011 at http://www.pbs.org/newshour/rundown/study-severe-food-allergies-more-common-among-children/.

Information on leaky gut syndrome is from "What is Leaky Gut?" on *Andrew Weil, MD* at http://www.drweil.com/drw/u/QAA361058/what-is-leaky-gut.html; and "Leaky Gut Syndrome: What Is It?" by Matt McMillen on *WebMD* at http://www.webmd.com/digestive-disorders/features/leaky-gut-syndrome.

Information on other factors in food intolerances is from "Food Allergy," on *Wikipedia* at http://en.wikipedia.org/wiki/Food_allergy; "Your Brain on Food," by Gary Wenk, June 21, 2011, *Psychology Today* at http://www.psychologytoday.com/blog/your-brain-food/201106/why-are-food-allergies-becoming-so-common; "Caesarean Section Babies May Have More Allergies and Diarrhoea," *Medical News Today,* October 21, 2004 at http://www.medicalnewstoday.com/releases/15292.php; "Allergies and the Breastfeeding Family," by Karen Zeretzke, *New Beginnings,* volume 15, issue 4, July–August 1998, p. 100, at http://www.lalecheleague.org/nb/nbjulaug98p100.html; "Chemical Hypersensitivity and the Allergic Response," *Ear, Nose, and Throat Journal,* volume 67, issue 1, January 1988 at http://www.aehf.com/articles/article36.html; "Roundup Linked to Global Boom in Celiac Disease and Gluten Intolerance," on *Sustainable Pulse,* Feb 19, 2014 at http://sustainablepulse.com/2014/02/19/roundup-linked-global-boom-celiac-disease-gluten-intolerance/#.UyoxQoWeb51; and "Global Pathfinder Report: Food Intolerance Products, Agriculture and Agri-Food Canada, International Markets Bureau Market Analysis Report," on *Agriculture Canada,* September 2012 at http://www.ats-sea.agr.gc.ca/inter/pdf/6256-eng.pdf.

CHAPTER 6

Information on stress from "Modern Life 'Too Stressful,'" July 21, 2005 at http://www.dailymail.co.uk/health/article-356542/Modern-life-stressful.html#ixzz33Adk3uqk; and "Can Stress Actually Be Good for You," on *NBC News* at http://www.nbcnews.com/id/15818153/ns/health-mental_health/t/can-stress-actually-be-good-you/#.UyzWHoWeb50.

CHAPTER 7

Information on organic toxins is from *Slow Death by Rubber Duck: How the Toxic Chemistry of Everyday Life Affects Our Health,* by Rick Smith and Bruce Lourie, Toronto: Random House, 2009. Information on inorganic toxins is from "Hazards of Heavy Metal Contamination," by Lars Järup, *British Medical Bulletin,* volume 68, issue 1, pages 167–182, at http://bmb.oxfordjournals.org/content/68/1/167.full; "Heavy Metal Detoxification" on *Life Extension Foundation for Longer Life at* http://www.lef.org/protocols/health_concerns/heavy_metal_detoxif ication_02.htm; and "Oxidative Stress," on *Wikipedia* at http://en.wikipedia.org/wiki/Oxidative_stress; "Lead Poisoning," *Wikipedia* at http://en.wikipedia.org/wiki/Lead_poisoning; and "Heavy Metal Detoxification," on *Life Extension Foundation for Longer Life* at http://www.lef.org/protocols/health_concerns/heavy_metal_detoxif ication_04.htm.

CHAPTER 8

Information on wellness and age management is from "Does Stress Cause Wrinkles and Gray Hair: Fact or Fiction?" by Vivian Diller, March 29, 2012 on *Psychology Today* at http://www.psychologytoday.com/blog/face-it/201203/does-stress-cause-wrinkles-and-gray-hair-fact-or-fiction.

CHAPTER 9

Information on children's health in general is from "Dextromethorphan," on *Drugs and Human Performance Fact Sheet, National Highway Traffic Safety Association* at http://www.nhtsa.gov/people/injury/research/job185drugs/dextr omethorphan.htm; "Vaccines," on *Wikipedia* at http://en.wikipedia.org/wiki/Vaccine; "Childhood Obesity," on *Government of Canada* at http://healthycanadians.gc.ca/kids-enfants/obesity-obesite/risks-risques-eng.php; "Child Obesity an Epidemic in Canada: Report," *Montreal Gazette,* March 28, 2007 at http://www.canada.com/montrealgazette/story.html?id=150adf76-6487-4779-abb9-e7d527a14f63; "Relationship Between Obese

Moms and Kids—Epigenetics, Home Environment or Both?" on *Nutrition Remarks*, May 10, 2013 at http://www.nutritionremarks.com/2013/05/10/relationship-between-obese-moms-and-kids-epigenetics-home-environment-or-both/.

Information on vaccines is from "Report an Adverse Event," on *Vaccine Adverse Event Reporting System* at https://vaers.hhs.gov/esub/index; "Vaccine Injury Compensation Program (VIPC)," on National Vaccine Information Center at http://www.nvic.org/injury-compensation.aspx; "Personal Stories," on *Vaccination Risk Awareness Network* at http://vran.org/personal-stories/; "Herd Immunity," on *Wikipedia* at http://en.wikipedia.org/wiki/Herd_immunity; "'Herd Immunity,' The Flawed Science and Failures of Mass Vaccination," by Suzanne Humphries, MD, on *International Medical Council on Vaccination*, July 5, 2012 at http://www.vaccinationcouncil.org/2012/07/05/herd-immunity-the-flawed-science-and-failures-of-mass-vaccination-suzanne-humphries-md-3/; "'Herd Immunity': The Misplaced Driver of Universal Vaccination," on *Vaccination Risk Awareness Network* at http://vran.org/about-vaccines/general-issues/herd-immunity/herd-immunity-the-misplaced-driver-of-universal-vaccination/; "Do Aluminum Vaccine Adjuvants Contribute to the Rising Prevalence Of Autism?" by L Tomlienovic and CA Shaw, Journal of Inorganic Biochemistry, November 2011, 105(11):1489–99, at http://www.ncbi.nlm.nih.gov/pubmed/22099159; "Responses to UBC Vaccine Paper a Problem for Free Scientific Inquiry and Expression," by Tom Sandborn on *Vancouver Courier*, Jan 30, 2012 at http://www.vancourier.com/opinion/responses-to-ubc-vaccine-paper-a-problem-for-free-scientific-inquiry-and-expression-1.375751; "Conflicts of Interest in Vaccine Safety Research," by Gayle DeLong in *Accountability in Research*, 19:65–68 at http://www.theoneclickgroup.co.uk/documents/vaccines/Conflicts%20of%20Interest%20in%20Vaccine%20Safety%20Research,%20Gayle%20DeLong.pdf; "Are Childhood Vaccines Dangerous?" by Dr. Andrew Weil on *Weil* at http://www.drweil.com/drw/u/QAA400067/Are-Childhood-Vaccines-Dangerous.html.

CHAPTER 10

Information on the mind-body connection from "Candace Pert," on *Wikipedia at* http://en.wikipedia.org/wiki/Candace_Pert; "Review of 'Molecules of Emotion,'" by Paul Trachtman, on *Smithsonian Magazine,* September 1998 at http://www.smithsonianmag.com/history/review-of-molecules-of-emotion-157256854/?no-ist; and "Candace Pert, 67, Explorer of the Brain, Dies," by John Schwartz, *New York Times,* September 19, 2013 at http://www.nytimes.com/2013/09/20/science/candace-pert-67-explorer-of-the-brain-dies.html.

CHAPTER 17

Information on children's health is from "Gut Flora," on *Wikipedia* at http://en.wikipedia.org/wiki/Gut_flora; and "Heavy Metal Detoxification," on *Life Extension Foundation for Longer Life* at http://www.lef.org/protocols/health_concerns/heavy_metal_detoxification_02.htm.

CHAPTER 19

Information on improving body composition through diet is from "Can a Food Diary Help You Lose Weight?" by Elaine Magee on *WebMD* at http://www.webmd.com/diet/features/can-food-diary-help-you-lose-weight; "The Power to Lose Like Never Before," on *Weight Watchers* at http://www.weightwatchers.ca/plan/index.aspx; "The Science of Eating Together," on *Food Tank,* July 4, 2013 at http://foodtank.com/news/2013/07/the-science-of-eating-together; "The Many Benefits of Breakfast," by Kathleen Zelman on *WebMD* at http://www.webmd.com/diet/features/many-benefits-breakfast; "Weight Control and Diet," on *University of Maryland Medical Center* at http://umm.edu/health/medical/reports/articles/weight-control-and-diet.

Information on improving body composition through exercise is from "Physical Exercise," on *Wikipedia* at http://en.wikipedia.org/wiki/Physical_exercise; "How to Get a Cardio Workout by Walking," on *For Dummies* at http://www.dummies.com/how-to/content/how-to-get-a-cardio-workout-by-walking.html; "Exercise: 7 Benefits of Regular Physical Activity," on *Mayo Clinic Healthy Lifestyle Fitness* at http://www.mayoclinic.org/healthy-living/fitness/in-depth/exercise/art-20048389; "What Types of Exercise Should I Do?" on *Osteoporosis Canada* at http://www.osteoporosis.ca/osteoporosis-and-you/exercise-for-healthy-bones/what-kind-of-activity-is-best/; "How to Find Your Target Heart-Rate Zone," on *For Dummies* at http://www.dummies.com/how-to/content/how-to-find-your-target-heartrate-zone.html; "Strength Training: Get Stronger, Leaner, Healthier," at *Mayo Clinic Healthy Lifestyle Fitness* at http://www.mayoclinic.org/healthy-living/fitness/in-depth/strength-training/art-20046670; "Strength and Flexibility Training" on *The Nutrition Source, Harvard School of Public Health* at http://www.hsph.harvard.edu/nutritionsource/strength-and-flexibility-training/; "Flexibility Training Section," on *Sports Fitness Advisor* at http://www.sport-fitness-advisor.com/flexibilitytraining.html; "Sample Flexibility Plan for Beginners," on Move! At http://www.move.va.gov/download/NewHandouts/PhysicalActivity/P33_SampleFlexibilityProgramForBeginners.pdf; and "Exercise and Weight Loss," on *WebMD* at http://www.webmd.com/diet/exercise-weight-control?page=2.

CHAPTER 20

Information on anaphylaxis is from "Facts + Advice," on *Anaphylaxis Canada* at http://www.anaphylaxis.ca/en/; "Severe Allergic Reaction (Anaphylactic Shock)," on *eMedicineHealth* at http://www.emedicinehealth.com/severe_allergic_reaction_anaphylactic_shock/article_em.htm; "Overview of Allergic Reactions," on *The Merck Manual Home Health Handbook* at http://www.merckmanuals.com/home/immune_disorders/allergic

reactions and other hypersensitivity disorders/overview of allergi c_reactions.html; "Food Allergies," on Health Canada at http://www.hc-sc.gc.ca/fn-an/securit/allerg/fa-aa/index-eng.php; and "The 8 Most Common Food Allergies," by Jeanette Bradley, May 16, 2014 *About.com Health: Food Allergies* at http://foodallergies.about.com/od/foodallergybasics/a/big_eight_fa. htm.

Information on diagnosing food intolerances is from "Food Allergies, or Something Else?" on *WebMD* at http://www.webmd.com/allergies/foods-allergy-intolerance; "Common Food Intolerances," on *Allergy UK* at http://www.allergyuk.org/common-food-intolerances/common-food-intolerances; "Elimination Diet Printable One-Sheet," on *The Dr. Oz Show,* Nov 12, 2013 at http://www.doctoroz.com/videos/elimination-diet-printable-one-sheet; "Food Sensitivities and Intolerances: Here's How to Do an Elimination Diet," by Bryan Walsh on *Precision Nutrition* at http://www.precisionnutrition.com/elimination-diet; "What's an Elimination Diet?" on *WebMD* at http://www.webmd.com/allergies/guide/allergies-elimination-diet; and "Antihistamines for Allergies," on *WebMD* at http://www.webmd.com/allergies/guide/antihistamines-for-allergies.

Information on managing food intolerances is from "How to Use a Rotation Diet," on *Allergy.org* at http://www.food-allergy.org/rotation.html; and "What is a Rotation Diet?" on *Rotation Diet Assistant* at http://www.rotationdietassistant.com/what-is-a-rotation-diet/.

CHAPTER 21

Information on stress is from "Cortisol: Its Role in Stress, Inflammation, and Indications for Diet Therapy," by Dina Aronson, *Today's Dietitian,* volume 11, issue 11, p. 38, at http://www.todaysdietitian.com/newarchives/111609p38.shtml; "Stress and Heart Health," on *American Heart Association* at http://www.heart.org/HEARTORG/GettingHealthy/StressManagem ent/HowDoesStressAffectYou/Stress-and-Heart-

Health_UCM_437370_Article.jsp; "Stress and Rheumatoid Arthritis,"
on *WebMD* at http://www.webmd.com/rheumatoid-arthritis/ra-
stress-response; "Psychological Stress and Cancer," on *National
Cancer Institute* at
http://www.cancer.gov/cancertopics/factsheet/Risk/stress; and Dr.
Sanjay Gupta, "Sugar," a segment on *60 Minutes,* aired on CNN April
1, 2012 and posted October 29, 2012 as "Sugar Exposé, 60 Minutes,
Dr. Sanjay Gupta" on *YouTube* at
https://www.youtube.com/watch?v=HezSlrJ1k7w.
Information on stress and control is from "5-HTT: The Gene for
Susceptibility to Depression?" on Davidson College at
http://www.bio.davidson.edu/courses/genomics/2003/mccord/5-
htt.html; "The Long-Term Costs of Traumatic Stress: Intertwined
Physical and Psychological Consequences," by Alexander C.
McFarlane, *World Psychiatry,* Feb 2010; 9(1): 3–10 at
http://www.ncbi.nlm.nih.gov/pmc/articles/PMC2816923/; "New
Study: Leaders Are Less Stressed Than Their Subordinates," by
Susan Adams on *Forbes,* September 27, 2012 at
http://www.forbes.com/sites/susanadams/2012/09/27/new-
study-leaders-are-less-stressed-than-their-subordinates/; "Poverty
Raises Levels of the Stress Hormone Cortisol: Evidence from
Weather Shocks in Kenya," by Johannes Haushofer, Joost de Laat, and
Matthieu Chemin, Oct 21, 2012 on *Dartmouth.edu* at
http://www.dartmouth.edu/~neudc2012/docs/paper_195.pdf;
"Religion Protects Against Stress, Study Suggests," on *CTV News,*
March 12, 2012 at http://www.ctvnews.ca/religion-protects-
against-stress-study-suggests-1.376003; and "Study: Non-Religious
People's Faith in Science Increases Under Stress," by Lindsay Abrams
on *The Atlantic,* Jun 6, 2013 at
http://www.theatlantic.com/health/archive/2013/06/study-non-
religious-peoples-faith-in-science-increases-under-stress/276583/.
Information on managing stress is from "Nine Ways Successful
People Defeat Stress," by Heidi Grant Halvorson on *Forbes,* Dec 23,
2102 at
http://www.forbes.com/sites/heidigranthalvorson/2012/12/23/ni
ne-ways-successful-people-defeat-stress/; and "Stop Expecting to
Change Your Habit in 21 Days," by Gretchen Rubin on *Psychology
Today,* Oct 21, 2009 at http://www.psychologytoday.com/blog/the-

happiness-project/200910/stop-expecting-change-your-habit-in-21-days.

CHAPTER 22

Information on managing toxic load is from "Top Three Sources of Toxic Exposures: Traffic, Personal Care and Plastic Products," by Joseph Mercola, May 15, 2013 on *Mercola.com* at http://articles.mercola.com/sites/articles/archive/2013/05/15/toxic-chemical-exposure.aspx; "Risk Of Heart Disease Increased By Long-Term Exposure To Fine Particles Of Traffic Pollution," on *Medical News Today,* April 21, 2013 at http://www.medicalnewstoday.com/releases/259314.php; "Fine Particulate Air Pollution and the Progression of Carotid Intima-Medial Thickness: A Prospective Cohort Study from the Multi-Ethnic Study of Atherosclerosis and Air Pollution," by Adar SD, Sheppard L, Vedal S, et al, PLoS Med, April 23, 2013, 10(4) on *PubMed* at http://www.ncbi.nlm.nih.gov/pubmed/23637576; "Chemicals from Personal Care Products Pervasive in Chicago Air," by Brian Bienkowski on *Scientific American*, Apr 30, 2013 at http://www.scientificamerican.com/article/chemicals-from-personal-care-products-pervasive-in-chicago-air/; "Lipsticks, Glosses Contain Toxic Metals: Report Children Should Not Play with these Products, Researcher Says," by Kathleen Doheny on *WebMD* at http://www.webmd.com/beauty/lips-smile/20130502/lipsticks-glosses-contain-toxic-metals-report?src=RSS_PUBLIC; and "Ten Retailers Urged to Pull Potentially Toxic Products," by Wendy Koch on *USA Today* at http://www.usatoday.com/story/news/nation/2013/04/09/retailers-products-toxic-chemicals/2067113/.

Information on naturopathic medicine is from "What is Naturopathic Medicine?" on *Canadian Association of Naturopathic Physicians* at https://www.cand.ca/index.php?78&L=0; "Definition of Naturopathic Medicine," on *American Association of Naturopathic Physicians* at http://naturopathic.org/content.asp?pl=16&sl=59&contentid=59; "Naturopathy: An Introduction," on *National Center for Complementary and Alternative Medicine* at http://nccam.nih.gov/health/naturopathy/naturopathyintro.htm; "Legal Status of Naturopathic Medicine," Bastyr University, http://www.bastyr.edu/academics/areas-study/study-naturopathic-medicine/about-naturopathic-medicine#Legal-Status. Information on detoxification is from "Chelation Therapy," on *Weil* at http://www.drweil.com/drw/u/ART03408/Chelation-Therapy.html; and "Metabolic Detoxification," on *Life Extension Foundation for Longer Life* at http://www.lef.org/protocols/metabolic_health/metabolic_detoxification_01.htm.

CHAPTER 23

Information on naturopathic scope of practice is from "Scope of Practice for Naturopathic Physicians: Standard, Limits, and Conditions for Prescribing, Dispensing, and Compounding Drugs," on College of Naturopathic Physicians of British Columbia at http://www.cnpbc.bc.ca/PDF-2010/SLC.%20Scope%20of%20Practice%20for%20Naturopathic%20Physicians%20Standards,%20Limits%20and%20Conditions%20for%20Prescribing%20Dispensing%20and%20Compounding%20Drugs%20%28Final%29%20corrections%2023.09.10.pdf. Information on supplementation is from *Drug-Induced Nutrient Depletion Handbook, 2ⁿᵈ Edition,* Hudson, OH: Lexi-Comp, 2001; *Encyclopedia of Nutritional Supplements,* Michael T. Murray, ND, Rocklin, CA: Prima Publishing, 1996 (http://doctormurray.com/); "About Us" and "Health Conditions," on *The Vitamin D Society* at http://www.vitamindsociety.org/about_us.php and http://www.vitamindcouncil.org/health-conditions/#; "New Vitamin D Guidelines," on *University of Calgary Faculty of Medicine,* July 14, 2010 at http://medicine.ucalgary.ca/about/vitaminD/Hanley; "New Study Will Address Vitamin D Dosages and Impact on Bone Health," on *UToday,* Jan 23, 2014 at http://www.ucalgary.ca/utoday/issue/2014-01-23/new-study-will-address-vitamin-d-dosages-and-impact-bone-health; "Coenzyme Q10 Evidence," on *Mayo Clinic Drugs and Supplements* at http://www.mayoclinic.org/drugs-supplements/coenzyme-

q10/evidence/hrb-20059019; "Coenzyme Q10 (CoQ10)," on *Weil* at
http://www.drweil.com/drw/u/ART03367/Coenzyme-Q10-
CoQ10.html; "Statin Drugs May Lower CoQ10 Levels," by Cathy
Wong, ND, June 27, 2008 on *About.com* at
http://altmedicine.about.com/od/consumerreviewsalerts/a/statins
_coq10.htm; "Magnesium Overview," on *University of Maryland
Medical Center* at
http://umm.edu/health/medical/altmed/supplement/magnesium;
"Selenium Overview," on *University of Maryland Medical Center* at
http://umm.edu/health/medical/altmed/supplement/selenium;
"Treatment of Depression: Time to Consider Folic Acid and Vitamin
B12," by A Coppen and C Bolander-Gouaille, on Journal of
Psychopharmacology, 2005 Jan;19(1):59–65 at
http://www.ncbi.nlm.nih.gov/pubmed/15671130;; "Vitamin B
(Folic Acid) Overview," on *University of Maryland Medical Center* at
http://umm.edu/health/medical/altmed/supplement/vitamin-b9-
folic-acid; "Zinc Fact Sheet for Health Professionals," on *National
Institutes of Health Office of Dietary Supplements* at
http://ods.od.nih.gov/factsheets/Zinc-HealthProfessional/ and
http://ods.od.nih.gov/factsheets/Zinc-HealthProfessional/#en72;
and "The Benefits of Vitamin C," by Kathleen M. Zelman on *WebMD*
at http://www.webmd.com/diet/features/the-benefits-of-vitamin-c.
Information on sleep is from "Sleep through the Decades," by Gina
Shaw on *WebMD* at http://www.webmd.com/sleep-
disorders/features/adult-sleep-needs-and-habits; "The Sleep
Solution Workbook," by G. Frank Lawlis on *Dr. Phil* at
http://www.drphil.com/assets/c/c0f3ab7356c5913f1a91dc7c7c34
7ecc.pdf; and "The Tranquiliser Recovery and Awareness Place," at
http://www.non-benzodiazepines.org.uk/withdrawa"l.html.
Information on water is from "Dehydration," on *Wikipedia* at
http://en.wikipedia.org/wiki/Dehydration; and "Water: How Much
Should You Drink Every Day?" Nutrition and Healthy Eating on Mayo
Clinic at http://www.mayoclinic.org/healthy-living/nutrition-and-
healthy-eating/in-depth/water/art-20044256.

CHAPTER **24**

Information on children's body composition is from "How to Calculate BMI for Children," on *Wikihow* at http://www.wikihow.com/Calculate-BMI-for-Children; "Nutrition for Children and Teens," on *HelpGuide* at http://www.helpguide.org/life/healthy_eating_children_teens.htm; "Healthy Eating Habits for Your Child," on *WebMD* at http://www.webmd.com/children/guide/kids-healthy-eating-habits; "Free Unstructured Play Is Essential For Children," on *Medical News Today,* October 9, 2006 at http://www.medicalnewstoday.com/articles/53699.php; "Student 'addiction' to technology 'similar to drug cravings,' study finds," by Andrew Hough on *The Telegraph,* April 8, 2011 at http://www.telegraph.co.uk/technology/news/8436831/Student-addiction-to-technology-similar-to-drug-cravings-study-finds.html; "Internet & Computer Addiction," on *HelpGuide* at http://www.helpguide.org/mental/internet_cybersex_addiction.htm ; "Top 10 Tips to Help Children Develop Healthy Habits," on *American Heart Association* at http://www.heart.org/HEARTORG/GettingHealthy/HealthierKids/HowtoMakeaHealthyHome/Top-10-Tips-to-Help-Children-Develop-Healthy-Habits_UCM_303805_Article.jsp. Information on children and toxic load is from "11 Toxic Chemicals Affecting Brain Development in Children," by Alice G. Walton on *Forbes,* Feb 15, 2014 http://www.forbes.com/sites/alicegwalton/2014/02/15/11-toxic-chemicals-afffecting-brain-development-in-children/; "Dirty Dozen List of Endocrine Disruptors," on *Environmental Working Group,* Oct 28, 2013 at http://www.ewg.org/research/dirty-dozen-list-endocrine-disruptors; and "Top Three Sources of Toxic Exposures: Traffic, Personal Care and Plastic Products," by Dr. Mercola, May 15, 2013 on *Mercola.com* at http://articles.mercola.com/sites/articles/archive/2013/05/15/toxic-chemical-exposure.aspx#_edn2. Information on children and sleep is from "How Much Sleep Do Children Need?" on *WebMD* at http://www.webmd.com/parenting/guide/sleep-children?page=2;

and "Backgrounder: Later School Start Times," on *National Sleep Foundation* at http://sleepfoundation.org/sleep-news/backgrounder-later-school-start-times.

Information on children and water is from "Health Issues: Heat Tolerance," on *Healthy Children* at http://www.healthychildren.org/English/health-issues/injuries-emergencies/sports-injuries/Pages/Heat-Tolerance.aspx; "U.S. Kids Don't Drink Enough Water," by Denise Mann on *WebMD* at http://www.webmd.com/children/news/20100924/u-s-kids-dont-drink-enough-water; and "Water Intake for Children Fact Sheet," on *Consortium to Lower Obesity in Chicago Children* at http://www.clocc.net/partners/54321Go/WaterIntake05-07.pdf.

ABOUT THE AUTHOR

Dr. Raj Jheeta has been a practicing naturopathic doctor in British Columbia, Canada since 1988. He studied biology at the University of British Columbia before transferring to the National College of Naturopathic Medicine in Portland, Oregon and graduating with a Doctoral Degree in 1987. When he began his private practice, he was the fifty-third Registered Naturopathic Doctor in Canada – a pioneer in a professional community that now exceeds 2,500 registered practitioners. He is a member of the College of Naturopathic Physicians of British Columbia and the British Columbia Naturopathic Association.

For the past 24 years, Dr. Jheeta has lectured internationally on naturopathic medicine on behalf of the Royal College of Physicians and Surgeons of Canada and the Royal College of the Physicians and Surgeons of the United States. His lectures on preventive medicine have addressed topics including heart disease, cancer, arthritis, drug-induced nutrient depletion, prescription drugs, herbal medicine interactions, and age management through nutraceutical medicines or functional foods. He is a specialist in preventive health care, wellness, and age management. He has been a primary care provider for several professional athletes and television personalities, and periodically provides health care tips to local media through television appearances and newspaper articles.

GLOSSARY

1. **Abdominal Rigidity** – an abnormally firm abdomen
2. **Abnormal Stools** – not subjectively considered normal or typical
3. **Acetaminophen** – a synthesized drug used to relieve pain and fever—called also paracetamol; see liquiprin, panadol, Tylenol
4. **Adiposities** – animal fat stored in the fatty tissue of
5. **Adrenal Gland** – either of a pair of complex endocrine organs near the anterior media border of the kidneys that secrete adrenal hormones
6. **Acid Reflux** – abnormal displacement of acid from the stomach to the esophagus
7. **Allopathic Medicine** – 1: a system of medical practice that aims to combat disease by use of remedies (as drugs or surgery) producing effects different from or incompatible with those produced by the disease being treated. 2: a system of medical practice making use of all measures that have proved of value in treatment of disease
8. **Allopathic Doctor** – one who practices allopathy
9. **Allopathy** – the prevailing form of medical practice to treat disease that uses remedies that have a different affect on the body than that of the disease
10. **Analgesia** – insensibility to pain without loss of consciousness
11. **Analgesic** – relating to, characterized by, or producing analgesia
12. **Anaphylactic Shock** – an often severe and sometimes fatal systemic reaction in a susceptible individual upon a second exposure to a specific antigen (as wasp venom or penicillin) after previous sensitization that is characterized especially by respiratory symptoms, fainting, itching, and hives
13. **Anaphylaxis** – hypersensitivity (as to foreign proteins or drugs) resulting from sensitization following prior contact with the causative agent
14. **Acne** – a disorder of the skin caused by inflammation of the skin glands and hair follicles; specifically, a form found chiefly in adolescents and marked by pimples especially on the face
15. **Antihistamine** – tending to block or counteract the physiological action of histamine

16. **Autoimmune Disease** – of, relating to, or caused by autoantibodies or T cells that attack molecules, cells, or tissues of the organism producing them
17. **Beryllium** – a steel-gray light strong brittle toxic divalent metallic element used chiefly as a hardening agent in alloys
18. **Body Mass Index (BMI)** – a measure of body fat that is the ratio of the weight of the body in kilograms to the square of its height in meters <a body mass index in adults of 25 to 29.9 is considered an indication of overweight, and 30 or more an indication of obesity
19. **Botanical Supplements** – derived from plants
20. **Breast Gland** – either of the pair of mammary glands extending from the front of the chest in pubescent and adult females of humans
21. **Caloric** – 1: a unit equivalent to the large calorie expressing heat-producing or energy-producing value in food when oxidized in the body 2: an amount of food having an energy-producing value of one large calorie
22. **Cancer** – 1: malignant tumour of potentially unlimited growth that expands locally by invasion and systemically by metastasis 2: an abnormal state marked by a cancer
23. **CBT** (cognitive behaviour therapy) – a type of talk therapy proven successful in treating various psychological conditions such as depression and anxiety
24. **Chelating Protocol** – methodology in which substances are used to manipulate, move, or eliminate compounds from the body
25. **Colonoscopy Study** – endoscopic examination of the colon
26. **Corticosteroid** – any of various adrenal-cortex steroids
27. **Cortisol (fight or flight response)** – a glucocorticoid $C_{21}H_{30}O_5$ produced by the adrenal cortex upon stimulation by ACTH that mediates various metabolic processes
28. **Detoxification** – to remove a harmful substance (as a poison or toxin) or the effect of such from
29. **DHEA** – Dehydroepiandrosterone - a weakly androgenic ketosteroid secreted by the adrenal glands that is an intermediate in the biosynthesis of testosterone and estrogens
30. **Diagnosis** – the art or act of identifying a disease from its signs and symptoms
31. **Digestive Stool Analysis** – evaluation of a stool sample for variances in digestive health
32. **Diagnostic** – using the methods of or yielding a diagnosis

33. **Differential Diagnosis** – in medicine, is essentially a process of elimination using various diagnostic tools to narrow down and determine the presence of a specific disease
34. **Eczema** – an inflammatory condition of the skin characterized by redness, itching, and oozing vesicular lesions which become scaly, crusted, or hardened
35. **Endocrine System (hormone regulation)** – the glands and parts of glands that produce endocrine secretions, help to integrate and control bodily metabolic activity, and include especially the pituitary, thyroid, parathyroids, adrenals, islets of Langerhans, ovaries, and testes
36. **Endocrine Function (hormones) Testing** – the method used to evaluate variances in endocrine function
37. **Enuresis** – involuntary urination, bed wetting, especially by children
38. **Fasting Blood Sample** – a blood sample taken most commonly after 12 hours of fasting
39. **Flatulent** – 1: marked by or affected with gases generated in the intestine or stomach 2: likely to cause digestive flatulence
40. **Food Preservatives** – something that preserves or has the power of preserving; specifically: an additive used to protect against decay, discoloration, or spoilage (a food preservative)
41. **Free T3 (Triiodothyronine)** – an iodine-containing hormone that is an amino acid derived from thyroxine
42. **Gastro Scope** – an endoscope for viewing the interior of the stomach
43. **Genetic Predisposition** – inherited or acquired predispositioning factor
44. **Heart Disease** - an abnormal organic condition of the heart or of the heart and circulation
45. **Hematology (blood) Tests** – a medical science that deals with the blood and blood-forming organs, blood test
46. **Homocysteine** – an amino acid marker that appears to be associated with an increased risk of cardiovascular disease when occurring at high levels in the blood plasma
47. **Hormone Disruptors** – chemicals or compounds that can alter the function of hormones
48. **Hypoglycemic** – a state of lower than normal blood sugar
49. **Immuno globulin-e** – is a class of antibody that plays an essential role in type 1 hypersensitivity (allergy)

50. **Ibuprofen** – a non-steroidal anti-inflammatory drug Used to treat fever and pain also known as Advil, Motrin
51. **Inflammation** – a local response to cellular injury that is marked by capillary dilatation, leukocytic infiltration, redness, heat, pain, swelling, and often loss of function and that serves as a mechanism initiating the elimination of noxious agents and of damaged tissue
52. **Insomnia** – prolonged and usually abnormal inability to obtain adequate sleep—called also agrypnia
53. **Irritable Bowel Syndrome (IBS)** – a chronic functional disorder of the colon that is of unknown etiology but is often associated with abnormal intestinal motility and increased sensitivity to visceral pain and that is characterized by diarrhea or constipation or diarrhea alternating with constipation, abdominal pain or discomfort, abdominal bloating, and passage of mucus in the stool — abbreviation IBS; called also irritable colon, irritable colon syndrome, mucous colitis, spastic colon
54. **LDL Cholesterol** – often referred to as the bad cholesterol low density lipoprotein
55. **Lesion** – an abnormal change in structure of an organ or part due to injury or disease; especially: one that is circumscribed and well defined
56. **Libido** – instinctual psychic energy that in psychoanalytic theory is derived from primitive biological urges (as for sexual pleasure or self-preservation) and that is expressed in conscious activity 2: sexual drive
57. **Locus** – a particular position, point, or place. (i.e. "it is impossible to specify the exact locus in the brain of these neural events")
58. **Menses** – blood and other matter discharged from the uterus at menstruation.
59. **Migraine** – a condition that is marked by recurrent usually unilateral severe headache often accompanied by nausea and vomiting and followed by sleep, that tends to occur in more than one member of a family, and that is of uncertain origin
60. **MRI Imaging** – magnetic resonance imaging used in the medical diagnostics
61. **Musculoskeletal** – of, relating to, or involving both musculature and skeleton
62. **Naturopathic Medicine (Naturopath)** – a distinct method of primary health care -an art, science, philosophy and practice of diagnosis, treatment, and prevention of illness. Naturopathic

physicians seek to restore and maintain optimum health in their patients by emphasizing nature's inherent self-healing process, the vis medicatrix naturae. This is accomplished through education and the rational use of natural therapeutics

63. **Naturopathic Doctor** – one who practices Naturopathy
64. **Nausea** – a stomach distress with distaste for food and an urge to vomit
65. **Nervous System** – the bodily system that in vertebrates is made up of the brain and spinal cord, nerves, ganglia, and parts of the receptor organs and that receives and interprets stimuli and transmits impulses to the effector organs—see autonomic nervous system, central nervous system, peripheral nervous system
66. **Nutrient Level Test** – various evaluation methods used to determine body levels of nutrients
67. **Oxycontin** – powerful narcotic classified analgesic
68. **Oxyneurine (Oxy-neo)** – a sweet crystalline quaternary ammonium salt $C_5H_{11}NO_2$ that was first isolated in beet juice and is used to treat homocystinuria and is also used in the form of its hydrochloride $C_5H_{11}NO_2 \cdot HCl$ as a source of hydrochloric acid especially to treat hypochlorhydria
69. **Palliation** – easing pain and suffering of a disease without removing the cause
70. **Palliative care** – health care that focuses on relieving pain and suffering of patients
71. **Palpation** – to examine by touch especially medically,
72. **Pesticides** – natural or chemically synthesized compounds used to control or eradicate pests, plant or animal
73. **Physical Medicine** – manipulation of the biomechanics of the body to diagnose or treat physical derangement a
74. **Prepubescent** – state of age and physical condition before puberty
75. **Preservative** – something that preserves or has the power of preserving; specifically: an additive used to protect against decay, discoloration, or spoilage (a food preservative)
76. **Prostate Gland** – a firm partly muscular partly glandular body that is situated about the base of the mammalian male urethra and secretes an alkaline viscid fluid which is a major constituent of the ejaculatory fluid - called also prostate

77. **Provocation Challenge** – evaluation method in which compounds are used to provoke the movement or elimination of various compounds from the body most often through the urine or stool
78. **Rheumatoid Arthritis** – an autoimmune disorder characterized by degenerative changes skeletal system particularly the joints, often involve pain and inflammation
79. **Steroid** – any of numerous natural or synthetic compounds containing a 17-carbon 4-ring system and including the sterols and various hormones and glycosides—see anabolic steroid
80. **Therapeutic (treating the problem)** – of or relating to the treatment of disease or disorders by remedial agents or methods – a therapeutic rather than a diagnostic specialty curative, medicinal (therapeutic activity of a drug) (therapeutic diets)
81. **Toxins** – inorganic or a colloidal proteinaceous poisonous substance that is a specific product of the metabolic activities of a living organism and is usually very unstable, notably toxic when introduced into the tissues, and typically capable of inducing antibody formation i.e. lead, mercury, benzene
82. **Triglycerides** – naturally occurring ester (complex of fatty acids and glycerol) that plays an essential role in the metabolism of adipose and glucose from the liver
83. **TSH (Thyroid Stimulating Hormone)** – a hormone that is secreted by the anterior lobe of the pituitary gland and stimulates the thyroid gland – abbreviation TSH – called also thyrotropic hormone, thyrotropin
84. **Ulcers** – a break in skin or mucous membrane with loss of surface tissue, disintegration and necrosis of epithelial tissue, and often pus (a stomach ulcer)
85. **Urinary Detoxification** – methods used to facilitate the excretion of toxins from the urine
86. **Urine Test (urine analysis)** – a diagnostic tool aimed at understanding metabolites found in urine samples to diagnose, evaluate and treat disease
87. **Vag Pac** – a concoction of herbs with properties toxic to cancer cells
88. **Vigor** – 1:active bodily or mental strength or force, 2: active healthy well-balanced growth especially of plants
89. **Visceral fat** - intra abdominal fat